This concise volume provides essential advice and guidelines for all those medical and allied personnel involved in the administration of radiation for diagnostic or therapeutic purposes. Legislation has been introduced to reduce patient radiation doses. There is thus a requirement for medical and other personnel to have received essential training in radiation protection.

This volume covers the background material required by those taking approved training courses in this area and summarises the core of knowledge which forms the basis of these regulations. It will therefore be an essential textbook for all staff who are concerned with diagnostic radiology, nuclear medicine or radiotherapy and who are about to undertake this training.

Radiation protection of patients

POSTGRADUATE MEDICAL SCIENCE

This important new series is based on the successful and internationally well-regarded specialist training programme at the Royal Postgraduate Medical School in London. Each volume provides an integrated and self-contained account of a key area of medical science, developed in conjunction with the course organisers and including contributions from specially invited authorities.

The aim of the series is to provide biomedical and clinical scientists with a reliable introduction to the theory and to the technical and clinical applications of each topic.

The volumes will be a valuable resource and guide for trainees in the medical and biomedical sciences, and for laboratory-based scientists.

POSTGRADUATE MEDICAL SCIENCE

Radiation protection
of patients

EDITED BY

R. WOOTTON

Professor and Director of Medical Physics,
Royal Postgraduate Medical School,
Hammersmith Hospital, London

Published in association with
the Royal Postgraduate Medical School
University of London by

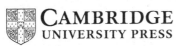

CAMBRIDGE
UNIVERSITY PRESS

Published by the Press Syndicate of the University of Cambridge
The Pitt Building, Trumpington Street, Cambridge CB2 1RP
40 West 20th Street, New York, NY 10011-4211, USA
10 Stamford Road, Oakleigh, Victoria 3166, Australia

First published 1993

A catalogue record for this book is available from the British Library

Library of Congress cataloguing in publication data

Radiation protection of patients / edited by R. Wootton.
p. cm. – (Postgraduate medical science series)
ISBN 0-521-42669-3 (pbk.)
1. Diagnosis, Radioscopic – Safety measures. 2. Radiotherapy – Safety
measures. I. Wootton, R. (Richard) II. Royal Postgraduate Medical
School. III. Series.
[DNLM: 1. Radiation Protection. WN 650 B1281]
RC78.3.R34   1993
616.07'57'0289 – dc20 92-49743 CIP

ISBN 0 521 42669 3 paperback

Transferred to digital printing 2004

KT

Contents

Acknowledgements

It is a pleasure to acknowledge the help and cooperation of a number of colleagues during the preparation of this text. In particular, I am grateful to:

- the Royal College of Radiologists for permission to reproduce their guidelines for doctors, entitled 'Making the Best Use of a Department of Radiology';

- the Director of the National Radiological Protection Board for permission to include material and to reproduce certain Figures from NRPB reports;

- the Bayeux City Authorities for special permission to reproduce a section of the eleventh century Bayeux Tapestry;

- Mr Doig Simmonds, the retired Head of Medical Illustration at the Royal Postgraduate Medical School, for his assistance with the artwork.

R. W.

Contributors

A. Bradley   Department of Medical Physics, Royal Postgraduate Medical School, Hammersmith Hospital, London W12 0NN, UK

K. C. Kam   Department of Medical Physics, Royal Postgraduate Medical School, Hammersmith Hospital, London W12 0NN, UK

M. J. Myers   Department of Medical Physics, Royal Postgraduate Medical School, Hammersmith Hospital, London W12 0NN, UK

M. Roddie   Department of Diagnostic Radiology, Royal Postgraduate Medical School, Hammersmith Hospital, London W12 0NN, UK

J. Shekhdar   Department of Medical Physics, Mount Vernon Hospital, Northwood, Middlesex HA6 2RN, UK

B. F. Wall   Medical Dosimetry Group, National Radiological Protection Board, Chilton, Oxon OX11 0RQ, UK

M. West   Department of Medical Physics, Royal Postgraduate Medical School, Hammersmith Hospital, London W12 0NN, UK

R. Wootton   Department of Medical Physics, Royal Postgraduate Medical School, Hammersmith Hospital, London W12 0NN, UK

Foreword

The primary purpose of this book is to present in a clear and comprehensive format the information concerning patient radiation protection that relates to the POPUMET Regulations introduced in 1988 (POPUMET stands for Protection of Persons Undergoing Medical Examination or Treatment). When it became a statutory requirement for a wide spectrum of health service workers to be familiar with POPUMET, the departments of Medical Physics and Diagnostic Radiology at the Royal Postgraduate Medical School instituted a teaching course to guide all those affected by this ruling through the legal and semantic complexities of the regulations. This teaching course, which is now repeated at regular intervals, has become so popular and created such a demand for further reference information available in an accessible and understandable format that it has become clear that a book such as this would be extremely valuable, not only as a useful complement to the Hammersmith (or any other) POPUMET teaching course, but also as a mini-work of reference in its own right.

Professor Wootton and his team of experts in various related fields have, I believe, succeeded brilliantly in their primary aim of synthesising all the material that is of importance in POPUMET into this clear and concise work. They have also, however, achieved a secondary purpose in that the information contained herein is, perforce, state of the art and it therefore serves an essential role in acting as an 'update' for professionals in the field. Radiation protection is a continually changing subject, particularly in view of the fact that our knowledge of the long term effects of ionising radiation remains incomplete. To keep up with current views in such a complex subject is an extremely difficult task for all those working in the field, but particularly so for those whose primary interest is in clinical matters rather than in physics. This work provides such individuals with a solution to their problem and, I believe, does so more succinctly and in a more readable fashion than any other available text. The importance of radiation protection is difficult to overestimate and nobody can be unaware of the intense interest in the subject at both national and international levels. Public awareness of radiation matters is increasing rapidly and the consumer magazine *Which?* has published a report on X-ray departments that concentrates heavily on this aspect of their performance. On the international scene, the International Commission on Radiological Protection has recently published guidelines for the reduction of exposure to levels below the current legal limits (ICRP Publication 60 – see Chapter 10), and this and other international initiatives all underline the need for professionals in the field to keep abreast of new developments.

Another important aspect of education in this area is the teaching of our future doctors. The medical students of today will, within a few years, be requesting radiological studies on many of their patients and, as future radiologists, cardiologists and other specialists, will be involved actively in the use of ionising radiation. We may need to work towards the introduction of the subject of radiation protection in the undergraduate medical curriculum and, given the existing pressures on that already overcrowded curriculum, a concise text such as this one may be the path to that goal.

Finally, it is worth pointing out the deliberate limitations of this book. In the interests of brevity and clarity it does not attempt to provide any great detail in the different areas it addresses. It does not, for instance, explain *how* to set up a quality assurance scheme in an X-ray department; rather it explains *why* such a scheme is necessary and provides the core of essential knowledge required for its successful implementation.

Professor Wootton and his team of authors are to be congratulated on their success in illuminating what, for many clinicians and for radiologists in particular, has been until now the murky and incomprehensible world of radiation protection.

D. J. Allison, BSc, MD, MRCP, FRCR
Professor and Director of Diagnostic Radiology,
Royal Postgraduate Medical School

Abbreviations

AED	Automatic exposure device
ALARA	As low as reasonably achievable
ALI	Annual limit on intake (of a radionuclide)
AP	Antero-posterior
ARSAC	Administration of Radioactive Substances Advisory Committee (of the Department of Health)
BIR	British Institute of Radiology
BSF	Backscatter fraction
CCTV	Closed circuit television
CRL	Crown–rump length
CT	Computed tomography
DNA	Deoxyribonucleic acid
DoE	Department of the Environment
DoH	Department of Health
DTPA	Diethylenetriamine-penta acetate
ED	Effective dose (formerly effective dose equivalent)
EC	European Community
HPA	Hospital Physicists' Association
HSC	Health and Safety Commission
HSE	Health and Safety Executive
HVT	Half-value thickness
ICRP	International Commission on Radiological Protection

IVU	Intravenous urogram
kVp	Kilovolts (peak)
LAT	Lateral
LET	Linear energy transfer
LLI	Lower large intestine
LMP	Last menstrual period
MAS	Product milliamp second
MRI	(nuclear) magnetic resonance imaging
NAIR	National Arrangements for Incidents involving Radio-activity
NHS	National Health Service
NRPB	National Radiological Protection Board
PA	Postero-anterior
PACS	Picture Archiving and Communication System
POPUMET	Protection of Persons Undergoing Medical Examination or Treatment
QA	Quality assurance
QALY	Quality-adjusted life year
QC	Quality control
RPA	Radiation Protection Adviser
RPS	Radiation Protection Supervisor
TAR	Tissue/air ratio
TLD	Thermoluminescent dosimeter
UK	United Kingdom
UNSCEAR	United Nations Scientific Committee on the Effects of Atomic Radiation

1

The need for radiation protection of the patient

R. WOOTTON

X-rays were discovered at the end of the nineteenth century and almost immediately employed in medical diagnosis. Enormous benefits to human health have resulted. The detrimental effects of ionising radiation were recognised early on, with the result that the history of radiation protection is very nearly as long as that of X-rays themselves. Until recently, however, the main focus of radiation protection in hospitals has been on the protection of the hospital staff rather than protection of the patient. The principal reason for this is that when a patient is irradiated during the course of a medical procedure it is the patient who, one hopes, benefits; in contrast, no benefit accrues to a member of staff who has been irradiated. In addition, it has been held as an article of faith for many years that the benefits to the patient far outweigh the risks. Why then should there be concern for radiation protection of the patient? There are several reasons.

First, radiation is damaging. As our knowledge of the long term effects of ionising radiation continues to grow, so, during periodic reviews of the available data, the risk factors have increased. The authoritative report from the International Commission on Radiological Protection (ICRP 60, 1991) has recently revised the risks upwards by a factor of three-to-fourfold. The bland assumption that the benefits outweigh the risks to the patient may not now be true in all cases, if indeed it ever was.

Second, medical irradiation is by far the largest man-made contribution to the radiation burden of the population of developed countries. Fig. 1.1 shows the situation in the UK, for example, where over 90% of the radiation dose from artificial sources is due to medical work. If radiation in population terms is undesirable, then it makes sense to tackle the largest component of the problem before it gets out

1

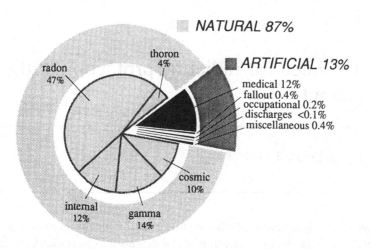

Fig. 1.1. The average annual radiation dose to the UK population is 2.5 mSv. Some 87% of the total is from natural radiation: half of the total is from radon exposure indoors. Medical exposure of patients accounts for about 12% of the total. All other sources – nuclear discharges, fallout, miscellaneous and occupational – account for 1% of the total (NRPB, 1989).

of control. For various reasons, very large sums of money have been spent on reducing the irradiation of the population resulting from the nuclear power industry. Whilst it should not be seen as a counter argument for so doing, relatively trivial sums spent on radiation protection of the patient would have a far bigger health impact.

Third, current practice in diagnostic radiology is undergoing continuous evolution in response to technological developments. For example, both the number of CT scanners, and the number of CT examinations, have shown an inexorable rise since the introduction of the technique in 1972 (see Table 1.1). A recent national survey has shown that while CT scans account for only about 2% of X-ray examinations in the UK, they result in 20% of the radiation dose due to medical X-rays (NRPB, 1991b).

Fourth, hospital X-ray equipment is often badly adjusted and badly used. The joint report of the National Radiological Protection Board and the Royal College of Radiologists stated that 'at least 20% of X-ray examinations currently carried out in the UK are clinically unhelpful in the sense that the probability of obtaining information useful for patient management is extremely low' (NRPB, 1990). Equipment quality assurance programmes, whilst much more common than, say, 20 years ago, are by no means universal.

Table 1.1. *Increase in the number of CT scanners operating in NHS hospitals since the introduction of the technique into clinical practice (NRPB, 1991a)*

	Number of operational scanners in NHS by year					
Manufacturer	1972	1978	1983	1985	1987	1989
GE	–	–	6	22	45	62
Siemens	–	–	10	21	35	50
Philips	–	–	5	13	18	23
Picker	–	–	2	7	9	11
Elscint	–	–	5	8	11	10
EMI	1	36	53	40	21	9
Technicare	–	–	3	3	3	3
Toshiba	–	–	1	3	4	4
CGR	–	–	–	–	1	1
Shimadzu	–	–	–	–	–	1
Meditech	–	–	1	1	1	–
Totals						
Scanners	1	36	86	118	148	174
Manufacturers	1	1	9	9	10	10
Models	1	3	19	30	36	39

Fifth, in the UK at least, there are continuing fiscal pressures on the National Health Service. The result is an undesirable situation in which medical equipment is neither kept up to date, nor supplemented or replaced by alternatives using non-ionising radiations where they exist.

Finally, it is the nature of low dose radiation injuries that they are apparently intangible. That is, they may occur at some considerable time after exposure and it is not possible to predict with certainty in which exposed individual the injury will occur. This has implications for radiation protection measures. What health service manager will pay more than lip service to a measure designed to reduce the number of deaths from cancer, when such deaths may occur at an unspecified time in the future (and probably in another health district) and when the numbers are so small as to be virtually undetectable against the natural incidence?

Against this background, both the EC and the UK parliament have introduced legislation aimed specifically at reducing patient radiation doses. In the UK, the Ionising Radiation (Protection of Persons Undergoing Medical Examination or Treatment) Regulations 1988, known colloquially as the POPUMET Regulations, were introduced. These require staff who, either clinically or physically, direct a medical

Table 1.2. *'Core of knowledge' as set out in the POPUMET Regulations*

Schedule	Regulations 5 and 6

Core of knowledge as to radiation protection of patients requisite for persons directing medical exposures

The following core of knowledge as to radiation protection of patients is that which a person physically directing medical exposures is expected to have acquired:

1. Nature of ionising radiation and its interaction with tissue.

2. Genetic and somatic effects of ionising radiation and how to assess their risks.

3. The ranges of radiation dose that are given to a patient with a particular procedure, the principal factors which affect the dose and the methods of measuring such doses.

4. The principles of quality assurance and quality control applied to both equipment and techniques.

5. The principles of dose limitation and the various means of dose reduction to the patient including protection of the gonads.

6. The specific requirements of women who are, or who may be, pregnant and also of children.

7. If applicable, the precautions necessary for handling sealed and unsealed sources.

8. The organisational arrangements for advice on radiation protection and how to deal with a suspected case of overexposure.

9. Statutory responsibilities.

For those clinically directing medical exposure, the following additional knowledge should be acquired:

10. In respect of the individual diagnostic and therapeutic procedures which the person intends to use, the clinical value of those procedures in relation to other available techniques used for the same or similar purposes.

11. The importance of utilising existing radiological information – films and/or reports – about a patient.

exposure to have received training in accordance with a Schedule to the Regulations, which is reproduced in Table 1.2. In addition, health authorities are required to keep an up to date register of their trained staff.

Following the introduction of the POPUMET Regulations, a number of approved training courses were established in the UK. The aim of this book is to include sufficient background material to encompass the required Core of Knowledge as set out in the Regulations.

Summary

Radiation protection of the patient is an important issue for a number of different reasons. These include the nature of ionising radiation itself, its long term effects on tissue, the size of the population dose from medical work, and certain economic factors.

Legislation in the UK requires staff concerned with ionising radiations to be properly trained.

References

ICRP 60 (1991). *1990 Recommendations of the International Commission on Radiological Protection*. ICRP Publication 60. Oxford: Pergamon Press.

NRPB (1989). *Radiation Exposure of the UK Population–1988 Review*. NRPB–R227. London: HMSO.

NRPB (1990). Patient Dose Reduction in Diagnostic Radiology. *Documents of the NRPB*. Vol. 1, No. 3. London: HMSO.

NRPB (1991*a*). *Survey of CT Practice in the UK. Part 1: Aspects of Examination Frequency and Quality Assurance*. NRPB–R248. London: HMSO.

NRPB (1991*b*). *Survey of CT Practice in the UK. Part 2: Dosimetric Aspects*. NRPB-R249. London: HMSO.

The Ionising Radiation (Protection of Persons Undergoing Medical Examination or Treatment) Regulations 1988. Statutory Instrument No. 778. London: HMSO.

2

Nature of ionising radiation and its interaction with tissue

R. WOOTTON

Atoms and molecules

All matter is made up of chemical elements. More than 90 elements occur naturally and there are about a dozen or so that have been produced artificially. The smallest portion of an element is the atom. Atoms themselves are very small: the diameter of an atom is about 10^{-10} m. One teaspoonful of water contains about 10^{23} atoms. Two or more atoms in combination form a molecule (e.g. H_2O).

Almost all of the mass of an atom is concentrated in its nucleus, which is positively charged. The atom as a whole is electrically neutral, since the positive charge on the nucleus is exactly balanced by one or more electrons, which are negatively charged particles. It is convenient to visualise the electrons as orbiting the nucleus. The orbits are relatively large, so that most of the space occupied by an atom is empty. If the nucleus of an atom had the diameter of a golf ball, the outermost electrons would be orbiting nearly a mile away.

Ionisation

The process of removing one or more electrons from an atom is called ionisation and an atom with one or more electrons missing is called an ion. Since there is a greater positive charge on the nucleus than the sum of the negative charges of the remaining electrons, the ion has a net positive charge. Not all forms of radiation are ionising. Visible light, for example, does not have enough energy to remove electrons from atoms.

6

Radioactivity

Most of the nuclei that occur naturally are stable and retain the same structure indefinitely. Some naturally occurring nuclei, and most artificially produced nuclei, are unstable: they are said to be radioactive because the change to a more stable structure is accompanied by the emission of radiation. This process is called radioactive decay. There are about 1700 known nuclides in all, of which the majority, about 1400, are radioactive. These are called radionuclides. Most are made artificially, but some, such as ^{14}C, ^{40}K and isotopes of uranium, thorium and radium, occur in nature. In the majority of cases, radioactive decay results in the emission of alpha particles, beta particles, or gamma rays. Note that the first two are forms of particulate radiation, while the latter are non-particulate i.e. electromagnetic radiation.

Electromagnetic radiation

Travelling waves (analogous to sound waves or water waves) in which the transverse oscillations are of electric and magnetic fields are known as electromagentic radiations. Light is a common example. The electromagnetic spectrum includes radiation ranging from long wavelengths (low frequencies), such as radiowaves, to short wavelengths (high frequency), such as X-rays. Visible light constitutes a small portion in the middle of the spectrum (Table 2.1).

Table 2.1. *The electromagnetic spectrum*

Type	Wavelength	Frequency	Energy
Radio (long wave)	1–100 km	3–300 kHz	
Radio (medium)	100 m	3 MHz	
Radio (short wave)	0.01 m	30 GHz	
Infra-red	700–10 000 nm	30–430 THz	
Visible			
(red)	700 nm	430 THz	
(blue)	400 nm	750 THz	
Ultraviolet	100–400 nm	750–3000 THz	3–12 eV
X-rays			
(soft)			1–10 keV
(hard)			100 keV
X-rays (from linear accelerator)			1–10 MeV
Gamma radiation			0.01–6 MeV

Gamma rays

Radioactive decay occurs when an unstable nucleus seeks a more stable structure. Sometimes this decay occurs in two stages: an alpha or beta particle is emitted first, but the nucleus still has too much energy for stability. The excess is emitted as a gamma ray, which follows very quickly after the original particle.

Gamma rays and X-rays are ionising because they have enough energy to remove electrons from atoms (visible light is not energetic enough). Gamma rays are more penetrating than alpha or beta particles (Fig. 2.1).

X-rays

Production of X-rays requires the excitation of an atom by a high speed particle. The particles used to produce medical X-rays are electrons that are accelerated at high speed towards a positively charged target, the anode. When the electrons strike the target they are slowed down abruptly. Some of the excess energy is emitted in the form of X-rays but the majority, some 99%, is converted to heat. The energy of the X-rays depends on the degree of interaction with the target atom, so there is a continuous spectrum of X-ray energy for a

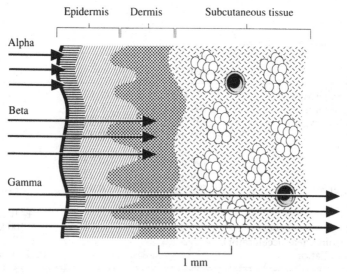

Fig. 2.1. Tissue penetration of alpha, beta and gamma radiations.

given incident electron energy. There may also be characteristic X-rays (Fig. 2.2).

Particulate radiations

In contrast to electromagnetic radiation, the particulate radiations are sub-atomic particles.

Alpha particles

A nuclide exhibiting alpha decay transforms to a more stable nucleus by emitting an alpha particle. An alpha particle is a nucleus of the element helium and consists of two protons and two neutrons. It therefore has two positive charges.

Alpha particles are emitted relatively slowly during decay. The low speed, relatively high mass and double positive charge all combine to make alpha particles highly ionising – that is, they tend easily to drag electrons out of atoms, thus transferring energy from the alpha particle

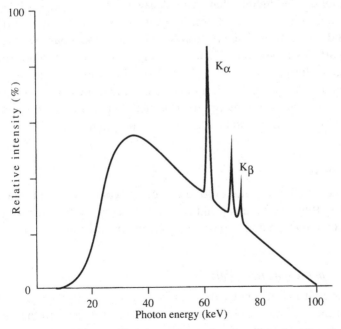

Fig. 2.2. The continuous X-ray spectrum from a tungsten target. The K characteristic X-ray lines are also shown.

to the electrons of the target material. As energy is transferred from the alpha particle, it slows down. The rate of energy transfer is higher in more dense materials. Thus alpha particles can travel several millimetres in air, but are absorbed extremely quickly in solids. The epidermis is usually thick enough to absorb all alpha particles emitted from radioactive materials.

Alpha decay occurs mostly in elements that are heavier than lead, such as uranium, thorium and plutonium. These radionuclides are not commonly used in medicine at present. Much more common are nuclides that emit beta particles.

Neutrons

Alpha decay is one way in which very heavy nuclei decay. Another method is by fission, either spontaneous or induced. In many fission processes, neutrons are released. Neutrons are uncharged.

Beta particles

Most radionuclides lighter than lead decay by beta emission. In the case of 'neutron-heavy' nuclides, a neutron is transformed into a proton and an electron. The electron is emitted as a beta particle.

Beta particles travel much faster than alpha particles. Because they are charged, they will interact with electrons in atoms that they come close to and cause ionisation, although not to the same extent as alpha particles will. A medium energy beta particle might travel for about 1 m in air, but in tissue would only travel for 1 or 2 mm.

Positrons

Certain radionuclides contain too few neutrons compared to the stable isotope i.e. they are 'neutron light' and can decay by transforming a proton into a neutron and a 'positive electron' or positron.

Other particulate radiations

As well as emitting beta particles, a nucleus can decay to a more stable state with the emission of electrons by two other processes. In the first, the nucleus imparts some of its energy to one of the orbital electrons. The electron is then ejected and the atom becomes ionised. The process is called internal conversion. Just as in the other cases of ionisation, an electron 'vacancy' is created, and this is filled quickly by an outer electron falling inward, until the vacancy is transferred to the outermost orbit of the atom. As the electrons move inwards, X-rays are emitted which can themselves cause further electrons to be ejected from the atom. These ejected electrons are known as Auger electrons.

Activity

The activity of a radionuclide is the number of nuclei decaying in unit time. The SI unit for activity is the becquerel (Bq), which is one decay per second. A source of 1 Bq is relatively small: the sizes of activities more commonly met are kBq or MBq i.e. 10^3 s^{-1} or 10^6 s^{-1}.

Note that one radioactive disintegration may result in the emission of more than one particle or photon. For this, and other, reasons there is no automatic relationship between amount of activity and degree of hazard.

Until recently, the unit of activity was the curie, which was defined as the number of nuclei decaying in a second in one gram of radium. This number is equal to 3.7×10^{10}, which is rather too large a unit for many applications. In medicine, activities of μCi or mCi were more common.

The activity of a given source is not constant, but changes (declines) with time as the number of undecayed nuclei in the source falls as a result of the decay process. The speed with which the activity in a source falls is measured by the half-life, which is the length of time required for the activity to fall by half. Thus after two half-lives, the activity will be reduced to one-quarter of its original value, after three half-lives to one-eighth, and so on. The half-life is characteristic of the particular radionuclide concerned e.g. ^{11}C has a half-life of 20 minutes, ^{99m}Tc 6 hours, ^{131}I 8 days, ^{125}I 8 weeks, ^{3}H 12 years.

Linear energy transfer

Alpha particles, beta particles, and gamma rays all cause ionisation and in this way give up their energy to the material they are passing through. Neutrons have no electric charge and do not therefore interact directly with electrons. However, they can cause ionisation indirectly, as a result of inducing radioactivity by being captured in a nucleus for example.

The linear energy transfer (LET) of a radiation is defined as the energy loss per unit of distance travelled. In general, a relatively slow moving alpha particle will cause more ionisation, and therefore have a higher LET, than a fast moving beta particle. It is usual to distinguish between alpha particles and neutrons, which are high LET radiations, and beta particles and gamma rays, which are low LET radiations. Auger electrons deposit their energy in a very small volume and therefore have similar effects to high LET radiation.

Absorbed dose

The activity of a radioactive source is the number of nuclei decaying per second. However, the activity gives no information about the biological effect of the radiation, since it does not, for example, indicate whether the disintegrations produce alpha, beta or gamma emissions. Biological effect is not easy to measure, but the starting point is the quantity of energy deposited by the radiation in unit mass of tissue. This is the absorbed dose, which is measured in units of grays (Gy). It is the fundamental dosimetric quantity in radiological protection work. One gray is equal to 1 joule of energy deposited in 1 kg of tissue. In radiation protection terms, one gray is a relatively large unit, milligrays or centigrays being more common in practice.

Until recently, the unit of dose measurement was the rad. The relationship between the two is: 1 Gy = 100 rad. Instrument scales calibrated in rad can therefore be conveniently relabelled in cGy.

Equivalent dose

The absorbed dose is the physical energy deposited in the target by the incident radiation. In order to measure biological effect, the absorbed dose is multiplied by a factor to take into account the nature of the radiation, since those with very high LET are relatively more damaging. This is the so called radiation weighting factor, formerly known as the quality factor. The equivalent dose in a tissue of type T, is thus:

$$H_T = D_{T,R} \cdot W_R$$

where $D_{T,R}$ is the absorbed dose due to radiation of type R and W_R is the radiation weighting factor. The majority of radiations encountered during clinical work are of similar LET values and have a weighting factor equal to unity. There is, therefore, a direct correspondence

Table 2.2. *Radiation weighting factors for the calculation of equivalent dose (ICRP 60, 1991)*

Type and energy range	Radiation weighting factor, W_R
Photons, all energies	1
Electrons and muons, all energies[a]	1
Neutrons, energy	
< 10 keV	5
10 keV to 100 keV	10
> 100 keV to 2 MeV	20
> 2 MeV to 20 MeV	10
> 20 MeV	5
Protons, other than recoil protons, energy > 2 MeV	5
Alpha particles, fission fragments, heavy nuclei	20

[a] Excluding Auger electrons emitted from nuclei bound to DNA.

between absorbed dose and equivalent dose. This is not always the case, however, and it should not be assumed automatically. Table 2.2 lists the radiation weighting factors in full.

The unit of equivalent dose is the sievert (Sv).

Effective dose

It is not usual in practice that a given irradiation will affect only a single organ. More commonly, several organs will receive radiation doses. In this situation it is convenient to be able to express the multiplicity of doses as a single value, which represents the hypothetical radiation dose that would have the same effect (risk) if it was *applied uniformly to the whole body*. This combined value is the effective dose (known formerly as the effective dose equivalent), and is also measured in sieverts. It is calculated by multiplying the equivalent dose in each organ, H_T, by a tissue weighting factor, W_T, and summing the result:

$$E = \sum H_T \cdot W_T$$

Table 2.3 gives the tissue weighting factors.

A sievert is a relatively large effective dose and lethal effects are produced in humans receiving doses in the range 1–10 Sv.

Table 2.3. *Tissue weighting factors for the calculation of effective dose (ICRP 60, 1991)*

Tissue or organ	Tissue weighting factor, W_T
Gonads	0.20
Bone marrow (red)	0.12
Colon	0.12
Lung	0.12
Stomach	0.12
Bladder	0.05
Breast	0.05
Liver	0.05
Oesophagus	0.05
Thyroid	0.05
Skin	0.01
Bone surface	0.01
Remainder	0.05[a]

[a] For the purposes of calculation, the remainder is composed of the following additional tissues and organs: adrenals, brain, upper large intestine, small intestine, kidney, muscle, pancreas, spleen, thymus and uterus. In those exceptional cases in which a single one of the tissues or organs in this category receives an equivalent dose in excess of the highest dose in any of the 12 organs for which a weighting factor is specified, a weighting factor of 0.025 should be applied to that tissue or organ and a weighting factor of 0.025 to the average dose in the rest of the remainder as defined above.

Absorption of ionising radiation in tissue

Absorption of ionising radiation in tissue takes place by a number of processes that depend on the characteristics of the absorbing material, on the energy of the incident radiation and on its nature e.g. whether the radiation is electromagnetic or particulate, and in the latter case, whether charged or uncharged.

Electromagnetic radiation

When electromagnetic radiation is absorbed in tissue, the ensuing biological effects are a consequence of the release of secondary charged particles. Production of these charged particles depends on the energy of the incident radiation and also on the composition of the tissue. Thus when X-rays or gamma rays with energies in the range

10 keV–100 MeV are absorbed in tissue, interactions will occur by photoelectric absorption, Compton scattering and pair production. Almost all of these processes depend on the atomic number of the absorbing material. Since bone has a higher effective atomic number (about 13) than soft tissue (about 7.5), this means that, particularly at low energies, the absorption in bone will be many times higher than that in soft tissue. This is the principle on which diagnostic radiology depends.

Charged particles

Charged particles (alpha and beta particles, electrons and protons) lose energy in tissue by collision and by radiative ('bremsstrahlung') processes. As charged particles slow down near the ends of their tracks, the ionisation per millimetre of tissue increases sharply. This is the so called Bragg peak.

Neutrons

Neutrons lose their energy by several mechanisms, including scattering, at energies above 100 eV. At low energies, hydrogen and nitrogen nuclei 'capture' so called thermal neutrons, thus rendering the nuclei radioactive.

Effects of radiation on cells

When ionisation occurs, one or more electrons are removed from atoms, bonds between atoms can be broken and the chemical constitution of the system is changed. Radiation can therefore damage cells through the process of ionisation.

One important type of damage caused by radiation is a change or break in the DNA of chromosomes i.e. a mutation. The damage caused in this way by radiation is random – the more radiation that passes through the cells, the higher the chance of damage occurring. Damage to the cell DNA can occur by a 'direct hit', or indirectly, due to ionisation of water molecules in the cell. Some damage to DNA can be repaired by the cell, while some may persist with long term consequences. Radiation effects that occur due to random events like this are called stochastic effects.

Effects of radiation on cell water

Since about 75% of the mass of the cell is water, more energy will be absorbed by water molecules than by any other molecule in the cell. One result of this is the formation of free radicals (e.g. H˙ and OH˙) which are reactive molecular fragments with unpaired electrons. The free radicals H˙ and OH˙ may combine with other free radicals, or they may react with other molecules in solution. For example, when two hydroxyl radicals combine, hydrogen peroxide (H_2O_2) is formed.

Direct and indirect action of radiation

When any form of radiation (X-rays or gamma rays, charged or uncharged particles) is absorbed in a biological material, there is the possibility that it will interact directly with the critical targets in the cells. This is the direct action of radiation. It is the dominant process when radiations of high LET (e.g. neutrons or alpha particles) are absorbed.

Alternatively, the radiation may interact with other atoms or molecules in the cell (particularly water) to produce free radicals that are able to diffuse far enough to reach and damage the critical targets. This is the indirect action of radiation.

Types of cell affected by radiation

The most likely effect of high radiation doses is that cells are sterilised i.e. cannot reproduce themselves. Many cells can be affected, but some parts of the body appear to be more sensitive to radiation than others. The reasons for this are complex, but are related partly to the turnover of cells in particular tissues. For example, in the lining of the gut there is normally a high rate of cell loss, which is continually being made good by newly divided cells. If the cells are sterilised by radiation, this replenishment can no longer take place, and eventually 'holes' appear in the gut wall. In a similar way, cells in the bone marrow that manufacture blood cells will show radiation damage more quickly than other body tissues. However, some tissues with low turnover of cells can be just as sensitive as those with high turnover and may show effects months or even years later.

Deterministic effects

High doses of radiation that damage many cells produce effects that can be related specifically to the radiation exposure. Some of these effects occur quite quickly, within days or weeks of exposure. Such effects include skin burns, various types of radiation sickness and damage to the lens of the eye. For each of these effects to occur, a minimum radiation dose or threshold has to be exceeded. Once the threshold is exceeded, the severity of the effect increases with the dose.

Effects of this type are called deterministic (formerly non-stochastic) i.e. the occurrence and severity of the effect is fairly predictable in any individual.

Stochastic effects

Low doses of radiation may affect only a few cells, or possibly only a single cell. Such damage may not cause any symptoms in the organism, and may be repaired subsequently. Any radiation damage that has occurred may not become apparent for years or even decades. It may then be difficult or impossible to link the observed abnormality with the exposure to radiation, since all the effects of low dose radiation can occur spontaneously or can be caused by other agents.

The approximate number of organisms that will be affected can be predicted if a large number are exposed to radiation, but the effect cannot be predicted with certainty for any particular individual. Effects of this kind are called stochastic i.e. random. There is no threshold for a stochastic effect and the probability of occurrence increases steadily as the dose increases.

Somatic and genetic effects

The stochastic effects of radiation can be classified as somatic or genetic: if radiation damage results in a disease or disorder in the organism itself, it is said to be somatic. However, if the damage appears not in the organism but in its descendants, then it is a genetic effect.

Summary

Ionising radiation may be electromagnetic, such as X-rays or gamma rays, or it may be particulate, for example neutrons, beta or alpha particles. Absorption of ionising radiation in matter is a complex process, and depends on the energy and nature of the radiation as well as the composition of the target.

Absorbed dose (Gy) measures the energy deposited in unit mass of tissue. *Equivalent dose* (Sv) takes into account the characteristics of the radiation. *Effective dose* (also Sv) is the hypothetical dose that would have the same effect if applied uniformly to the whole body.

At high doses of radiation, deterministic effects occur: there is a definite threshold above which the severity of the effects increase with the dose. At low doses there may be stochastic effects: these do not have a threshold for occurrence and are difficult to predict in a particular individual.

References

ICRP 60 (1991). *1990 Recommendations of the International Commission on Radiological Protection*. ICRP Publication 60. Oxford: Pergamon Press.

3

Genetic and somatic effects of ionising radiation and how to assess their risks

M. J. MYERS

Introduction

The interaction of radiation with tissue implies some alteration and consequently some element of *damage* to the tissue. This damage may act by weeding out unhealthy cells in the body, in which case the radiation has a beneficial effect (this is known as hormesis and has the same rather nebulous clinical standing as homeopathy). However, in the overwhelming majority of cases the radiation tends to be harmful.

High doses of radiation, for example, those from a nuclear reactor accident or nuclear bomb, have rather gross effects such as death from central nervous system radiation sickness. These effects are not relevant to medical diagnosis, where diagnostic doses of the order of one thousandth or less, relative to therapeutic irradiation, are administered. They may be pertinent to radiotherapy however. Biological effects may be divided into a number of categories according to the way they affect different functions of the body and the different ways they take effect. A number of terms like 'genetic' and 'somatic', 'stochastic' and 'deterministic' and 'acute' or 'chronic' have been used to describe the radiation effects.

Mechanism of damage

The process of damage involves the transfer of very small quantities of energy from the radiation to the cell. Individual events affecting a few cells would not, at first glance, be expected to have much influence on the body. (The average natural background radiation dose of 2.5 mSv is equivalent in energy terms to a table tennis ball dropped on a person from a height of 10 m). And yet, if the right target is struck and the right chain of events is triggered off, the result could be death from cancer decades later.

Although the basis of the sensitive trigger effect and the exact mechanism of damage are unknown, a working model is that ionisation causes damage to a cell by creating double-strand breaks in DNA that are not repaired properly. For this to occur, the destructive effects of different kinds of radiation are related to the *pattern* of ionisations in the vicinity of the DNA material. At just the right spacing of bursts of ionisations, both the chains of the DNA molecule can be split at the same time and recombine incorrectly (see Fig. 3.1). This is most likely to occur when high energy particles slow down or when low energy particles appear near the nucleus and the spacing between the bursts of ionisation is reduced. For destruction of the other large molecules in cells, such as enzymes and proteins, very large doses are required. Thus a dose equivalent to tens of grays is needed for substantial

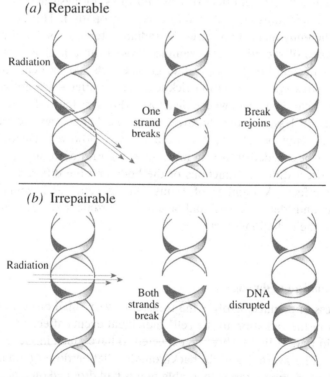

Fig. 3.1. Damage to DNA may be (*a*) temporary and repairable or (*b*) it may be irrepairable and have serious long lasting effects.

ionisation of respiratory enzymes and alteration of cell function. One reason for this is that the body has a large reserve of these molecules.

Genetic and somatic damage due to radiation

Radiation is introduced into the body as extremely small parcels of energy. As such, it has effects at the level of individual cells of the body. Usually the only component of importance that is changed or damaged is the DNA of the nucleus of cells. If the DNA is contained within a germ (reproductive) cell the change in function may be passed on through the developing embryo to a live child. This is the *genetic* effect of radiation, an example of which is the production of a child with Down syndrome. If other DNA molecules are damaged, this may trigger off a series of changes in a population of cells and thus an organ or particular function of the body is affected. This would constitute a *somatic* effect, examples of which are skin reddening and cataract formation.

If changes in genetic material (chromosomes) occur because of radiation damage to the egg or the sperm, then a descendant rather than the person irradiated may show an abnormality (Fig. 3.2). The inherited diseases resulting from the genetic damage add to those produced by many other factors (such as chemical or spontaneous mutation). Studies of the incidence of genetic disease in large populations show that 9% of liveborn have one form or another of genetic abnormality, and that about 0.6% of these abnormalities are chromosomal diseases.

No significant increase in the frequency of abnormalities in the children of atomic bomb survivors compared with unaffected individuals has been seen and there also may be other associations between the incidence of spontaneous abortion and maternal irradiation history. The association between the incidence of Down syndrome, a mainly genetic abnormality, and radiation exposure has not been found to be significant. However, after irradiation of the fetus, its subsequent development of cancer is more likely. With a low or insignificant number of genetic abnormalities from human studies on which to base firm conclusions, the results of animal experiments have been extrapolated to predict the small increases in these abnormalities in humans, as discussed below.

In the same way that the genetic effects of radiation superimpose on naturally occurring disease, so somatic effects, mainly expressed in the

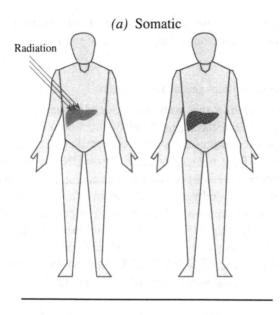

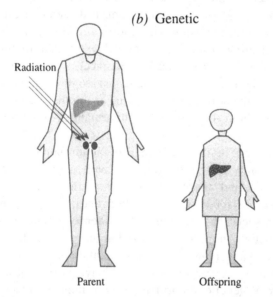

Fig. 3.2. Radiation damage may be (*a*) somatic, affecting the individual irradiated or (*b*) through damage to germ cells, may result in genetic effects in subsequent generations.

form of excessive cancer incidence or mortality, are superimposed on naturally occurring cancer.

At low doses, such effects as acute radiation sickness involving the central nervous, gastrointestinal and bone marrow systems, skin burns, hair loss, infertility and cataract formation may be ignored.

Stochastic and deterministic effects

Radiation is a fundamentally random process; it can never be predicted exactly which cells in the body will be affected. However, it would be natural to expect that at high doses more cells might be affected and therefore more damage might be done than at low doses – the severity of the damage and/or the frequency of the damaging events will depend on the dose. It is also conceivable that changes might not occur until a threshold dose is reached i.e. not enough cells are permanently transformed to produce a noticeable effect. Two terms have been introduced to classify the damage due to radiation through two different processes. These terms are difficult to conceptualise but are useful in separating different effects and legislating to minimise their incidence.

Those effects that occur only after a minimum dose has been received and then result in increasing severity of damage and increasing number of transformed cells are called *deterministic* effects (Fig. 3.3(a)). Formerly they were known as non-stochastic, and since the word stochastic means random, the term non-stochastic can be taken to mean that the effects are not random but quite predictable. To a certain degree the effects can be largely predicted for a particular individual from the dose received. Examples of deterministic effects are skin erythema and ulceration.

In contrast, those effects that take place even at very low dose levels, and where the number of cells transforming increases with increasing dose, are called *stochastic* effects (Fig. 3.3(b)). These are chance events, as seen from the name, and by definition cannot be predicted accurately in any one individual and can be quantified only in terms of probabilities derived from a study of a large, affected population. While the probability of their occurrence is a function of dose, their effect on an individual does not vary. Thus the *probability* of the radiation inducing leukaemia in a person increases with increasing radiation. There is no variation in effect as there is with determin-

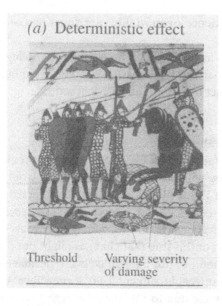

(a) Deterministic effect

Threshold   Varying severity
                 of damage

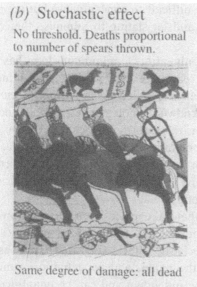

(b) Stochastic effect

No threshold. Deaths proportional
to number of spears thrown.

Same degree of damage: all dead

Fig. 3.3. Radiation damage following high doses *(a)* is deterministic and fairly predictable. In contrast, *(b)* at low doses it is stochastic or random in effect. (Section of the eleventh century Bayeux Tapestry reproduced by special permission of the Bayeux City Authorities.)

istic events i.e. the effect is the same leukaemia (or the same death) whatever the dose level.

Cancer production affecting the breast, lung, blood, thyroid and other organs are the main (stochastic) effects of radiation. The mechanism involves transformation of the cell to increase its malignant potential with consequent development, after a latency period, of a detectable cancer. The three steps of initiation, promotion and progression ascribed to general development of cancer have been associated with radiation-induced tumours, though these concepts are not fully explained (Fig. 3.4).

This discussion implies that, for a deterministic effect, if the threshold is never exceeded when working with or subjected to radiation, then essentially no radiation danger exists. It is, therefore, very important to establish the level of threshold dose in order to keep below it. For stochastic damage all that can be done is to minimise the dose in order to minimise the problems.

Risks

In examining the effects of radiation, three populations are of interest because of the different ways they are exposed: patients, workers and the public (with the developing embryo as a special case of the innocent patient).

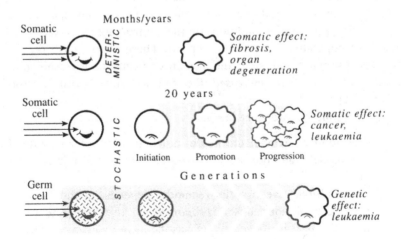

Fig. 3.4. The long term time course and results of deterministic and stochastic effects on somatic and germ cells.

Table 3.1. *Human fatal cancer risk, age and sex averaged, for high doses and dose rates (NRPB, 1988)*

Source of estimate	Population	Risk of fatal cancer[a] (per mSv)
UNSCEAR (1977)	All	2.5×10^{-5}
UNSCEAR (1988)	Workforce (age 25–64)	4×10^{-5} to 6×10^{-5}
	General population (all ages)	4×10^{-5} to 5×10^{-5}

[a] Based on the absolute-risk projection model.

Three risks from the low level radiation used in diagnosis are of concern:

1 The risk of genetic damage passed on as inherited disease.
2 The risk of malformation or cancer to the fetus of an irradiated pregnant woman.
3 The risk of development of cancer, or death from cancer, induced by radiation.

UNSCEAR (the United Nations Scientific Committee on the Effects of Atomic Radiation) has recently reconsidered the data on three populations in which dose–effect relations have been established. These populations are the atomic bomb survivors in Japan, the group of patients once treated for ankylosing spondylitis and the Marshall Islanders exposed to radiation in atomic bomb tests. New factors such as the effect of weather conditions on the neutron dose received by the Japanese populations have been applied. These factors have reduced the dose estimates and, since the incidence of cancer has remained the same, have therefore *increased* the risk associated with radiation (Table 3.1).

Two risk models are considered:

1 The additive or absolute model is independent of base rate. In this model, radiation adds a fixed amount to the natural incidence.
2 The multiplicative or relative model depends on the base rate because radiation adds a *proportion* of the base rate to the natural cancer incidence. It reflects the higher incidence of cancer at the end of life-span resulting in a higher estimate of the number of cancers. Currently this is the favoured model.

Both models are illustrated in Fig. 3.5.

Since, for diagnosis, both dose and dose rate are reduced compared with the atomic bomb conditions, a number of dose rate reduction factors have been applied by various official committees. These reduction factors are shown in Table 3.2: their values range from two to ten. Taking this into account, the risk factors for protection work are as shown in Table 3.3.

Risk of cancer

Unlike the link between irradiation and genetic abnormalities, the relation between irradiation and cancer has been established and quantified as a function of dose. A straight-line relationship between dose and effect without threshold (one that goes through the origin) is usually employed. This is the so-called linear model. Risk figures have been established for cancers of different organs or tissues and are listed in Table 3.4. The assumption of a straight-line relationship may however be incorrect. Since the experimental data are known only for high doses, the curves may actually look like those illustrated in Fig. 3.6.

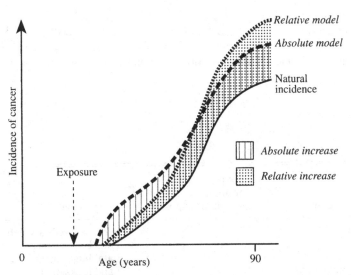

Fig. 3.5. Two models for the increased incidence of cancer following irradiation. The natural incidence, which rises steeply with age, is shown as a solid line. The *absolute model* predicts a constant increase above the baseline; the *relative model* predicts a proportional increase.

Table 3.2. *Dose rate reduction factors*

Source of estimate	Reduction factor
UNSCEAR (1977) (linear response model)	2
UNSCEAR (1986)	< 5
UNSCEAR (1988)	2–10 (10 for ^{131}I in the thyroid)
NRPB (1988)	3

Table 3.3. *Risk factors*

	Risk factor[a] (per mSv)	Risk
Fatal cancers		
IRCP26 (1977)	1.25×10^{-5}	(1 in 80 000)
ICRP60 (1991)	4×10^{-5}	
	to 5×10^{-5}	(1 in 20 000 to 1 in 25 000)
Hereditary defects		
Two generations	0.4×10^{-5}	(1 in 250 000)
All generations	0.6×10^{-5}	
	to 1×10^{-5}	(1 in 100 000 to 1 in 170 000)
Total (weighted to allow	5×10^{-5}	(1 in 14 000
for non-fatal cancer)	to 7×10^{-5}	to 1 in 20 000)

[a] The higher risk factors apply to workers and the lower to members of the public.

Table 3.4. *Organ risk factors*

Organ or tissue	Risk per mSv per million individuals exposed	Consequence
Gonads	10	Serious hereditary defect
Breast	2	Fatal breast cancer
Lung	8.5	Fatal lung cancer
Red bone marrow	5	Fatal leukaemia
Thyroid	0.8	Fatal thyroid cancer
Other tissues e.g. stomach, LLI, liver	5	Fatal cancer

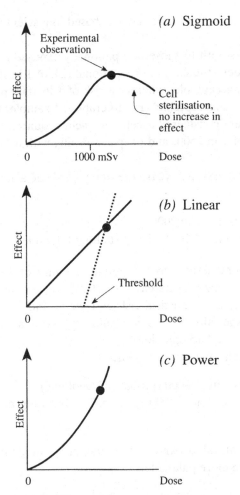

Fig. 3.6. Radiation effects at low doses have to be predicted from experimental observations at high doses using a model. Common models assume the response to be (*a*) sigmoidal, (*b*) linear, with or without a threshold, or (*c*) a power law.

Risks in general and from radiation

Risk is associated with all human activities and can occur over a wide range between what is clearly acceptable and what is clearly unacceptable; limits must be set in the grey area between the extremes. These limits are often governed by politics (e.g. cost, priorities etc.), pragmatism (need to work, travel etc.) and social acceptability (e.g.

society's view of smoking), rather than advice based on scientific evidence.

The acceptability of risks both to those occupationally exposed and to the general public has been studied. An occupational risk of 1 in 100 per year was considered unacceptable, whereas a risk of 1 in 1000 per year was thought to be 'not unacceptable' (i.e. tolerable). Examples of high risk occupations that are considered acceptable include quarrying, with a fatal accident rate of 1 in 2500, and deep sea fishing with a 1 in 1000 risk.

For radiation work at 50 mSv per year, the annual risk of a fatal cancer is as follows:

> based on 'old' dosimetry: 1 in 2000
> based on revised dosimetry: 1 in 500 i.e. just about tolerable

For annual risks of a general nature to the public, a figure of 1 in 10 000 was considered unacceptable, whereas 1 in 100 000 was probably acceptable. This, of course, is a statistical risk and for an individual member of the public (especially after some publicity) even a low probability risk may not be at all acceptable.

For irradiation of the public at 1 mSv per year:

> the old risk estimate is 1 in 100 000 (probably acceptable)
> the new risk estimate is 1 in 20 000 (reasonable, but only as a limit)

The unavoidability of a natural background of the order of 2 mSv makes the new risk estimate more palatable.

Proposals for future dose limits

Current thinking, as outlined in ICRP 60 (1991) but not yet enshrined in any UK or European legislation, is that it would be prudent to keep the *average* effective dose to 20 mSv per year, where the average is calculated over a period of five years. If the average was consistently 20 mSv per year, this would yield a lifetime risk of about 5% for fatal cancer, which is barely acceptable. In addition, there are risks of non-fatal cancer, or of severe hereditary effects, amounting to about 1%.

Practical schemes might be:

for workers:
20 mSv per year averaged over five years (and not exceeding 50 mSv in any one year)
500 mSv per year to the skin or the hands and feet

for the public:
1 mSv per year averaged over five years
50 mSv per year to the skin

Following the revised dosimetry rather strictly, gives:

> annual dose to worker set at 20 mSv with classification at 7 mSv
> annual dose to general public of 1 mSv (cf. natural background of 2.5 mSv per year)
> limit to controlled area set at the discretion of the RPA, who will ensure that dose limits to workers are not exceeded

There should be no problems associated with an annual dose limit of 20 mSv, especially when averaged over some years, but keeping the public dose below 1 mSv may necessitate changes in diagnostic and therapeutic X-ray and nuclear medicine workpractices.

Radiation doses from natural sources

The total radiation dose from natural sources is about 2 mSv per year (Table 3.5). Comparing that with the approximate doses of 0.05 mSv for a chest X-ray, 1.4 mSv for an abdominal X-ray, or 4 mSv for a radioisotope bone scan, puts the cost, in terms of the radiation dose, of obtaining medical information more in perspective.

Comparison with other risks

For comparison, Table 3.6 shows activities that carry a 1 in 10 000 risk.

Summary

Ionising radiation has a wide range of effects on the body in terms of time span (immediate or long term), of generations affected (present and future), of severity (all or nothing, or graded) and of thresholds of effect (stochastic and deterministic).

Legislation can prevent deterministic effects by reducing doses to

Table 3.5. *Annual exposure of the UK population from all sources of radiation (NRPB, 1989)*

Source	Dose rate (μSv/year)
Natural	
Cosmic radiation	250
Terrestrial gamma rays (uranium & thorium)	350
Internal irradiation (^{40}K, ^{14}C, ^{210}Pb)	300
Radon and its decay products	1200
Thoron and its decay products	100
Sub-total (natural)	2200
Artificial	
Medical	300
Miscellaneous	10
Fallout	10
Occupational	5
Discharge	< 1
Sub-total (artificial)	325
Total	2500

Table 3.6. *Activities carrying a one in 10 000 risk of death*

Whole body exposure to 2 mSv of ionising radiation.

Smoking 150 cigarettes (*smoking 20 cigarettes a day for 20 years, a total of 150 000, gives a 1 in 10 chance of dying*).

Travelling 5000 miles by car (*a five-mile drive to work each day is equivalent, in terms of risk of death over a week, to receiving 2 mSv of radiation in that week. A total of 10 000 miles a year for ten years gives a 1 in 500 chance of death*)

Travelling 25 000 miles by passenger aircraft (*this is the risk from increased radiation exposure; making ten transatlantic journeys gives a 1 in 5000 chance of dying through crashing, fire etc.*)

Rock climbing for 2.5 hours.

Canoeing for 10 hours.

Working in a typical factory for four years (*through being exposed to the risk of an occupational accident at work*).

Being a woman aged 18 years for 4 months (*1 in a million 18-year-old women die each day from any cause of death*).

Being a man aged 30 or a woman aged 35 years for 1 month.

Being a man aged 63 or a woman aged 71 years for 1 day.

sub-threshold levels, but stochastic effects can be minimised only by minimising radiation exposure in general.

Risks from exposure to low levels of radiation are difficult to estimate accurately. Present knowledge indicates that the risks of total cancer are of the order of 5% per sievert (i.e. a risk of about 1 in 20 000 for each mSv).

References

ICRP 26 (1977). *Recommendations of the International Commission on Radiological Protection.* ICRP Publication 26. Oxford: Pergamon Press.

ICRP 60 (1991). *1990 Recommendations of the International Commission on Radiological Protection.* ICRP Publication 60. Oxford: Pergamon Press.

NRPB (1988). *Health Effects Models Developed from the 1998 UNSCEAR Report.* NRPB-R226. London: HMSO.

NRPB (1989). *Radiation Exposure of the UK Population–1988 Review.* NRPB-R227. London: HMSO.

UNSCEAR (1977). *Sources and Effects of Ionizing Radiation.* Report to the General Assembly, with Annexes. New York: United Nations.

UNSCEAR (1986). *Genetic and Somatic Effects of Ionizing Radiation.* 1986 Report to the General Assembly with annexes. New York: United Nations.

UNSCEAR (1988). *Sources, Effects and Risks of Ionizing Radiation.* 1988 Report to the General Assembly, with annexes. New York: United Nations.

4

Radiation doses. The ranges of radiation dose that are given to a patient with a particular procedure, the principal factors that affect the dose and the methods of measuring such doses

M. J. MYERS

National radiation surveys

Surveys have been carried out, both in the UK and abroad, in which the radiation doses involved in dozens of X-ray procedures on millions of patients have been analysed. A limited set of such procedures is discussed here. The examinations have been chosen either because they contribute the greatest radiation dose to the population as a whole or because they are amongst those most frequently employed.

In a survey carried out in the UK by the National Radiological Protection Board (NRPB, 1986; Shrimpton *et al.*, 1986) a series of ten types of X-ray examinations that contribute nearly 90% of the collective radiation dose of the UK was selected. These examinations were divided into two classes: 'simple' such as an X-ray of the abdomen (Fig. 4.1) and 'complex' such as an IVU (Fig. 4.2). In general the complex examinations were associated with a greater dose to the patient.

Similar surveys for the field of nuclear medicine have also been carried out. These have given information about the frequency with which different nuclear medicine procedures are performed. From one such survey a list of ten imaging procedures, covering about 70% of the total number performed, was drawn up (Wall *et al.*, 1985).

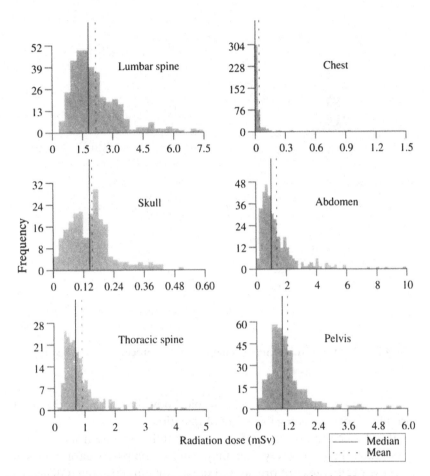

Fig. 4.1. Radiation doses from six of the most common 'simple' X-ray procedures. Each histogram shows the number of times a particular dose was recorded for a procedure, the mean and median doses and the range of doses (NRPB, 1986).

Effective dose

The radiation dose arising from X-radiation entering the body from an external source is most easily measured as a surface (skin) dose. However, since it is individual internal organs that are the targets of the X-rays, it is better to consider the organ dose. Because the risk to the individual is the result of an effective summation of doses to all the organs, the whole body dose may be the best way of comparing doses between procedures. For nuclear medicine, where all parts of the body

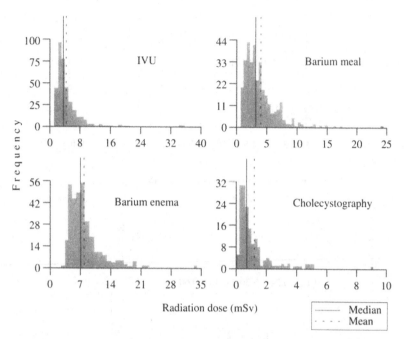

Fig. 4.2. Results for four common 'complex' X-ray procedures (NRPB, 1986).

are affected to some extent, the whole body dose is again the most useful way of expressing the effect of radiation.

It is difficult to express simply but accurately the dose from different procedures in such a way that they can be compared easily. This is because of the range of organs and tissues that are examined diagnostically, each with its own sensitivity and each receiving a different proportion of the total body dose. To take account of this, the 'effective dose' or ED is normally used as a simple, single figure index of the dose. To calculate the ED, a 'weighting factor' is ascribed to each organ. This weighting factor is based on the risk factor per mSv per million population (Fig. 4.3).

The weighting factor is expressed as the fractional risk to the organ in question compared with the total risk factor for uniform whole body irradiation. A primary list of radiosensitive organs is defined, and includes the gonads, bone marrow, colon, lung and stomach. Thus the thyroid, with a relatively low risk, is given a weighting factor of 0.05, while the higher sensitivity of the gonads to radiation is expressed by a weighting factor of 0.20. For each type of examination, additional

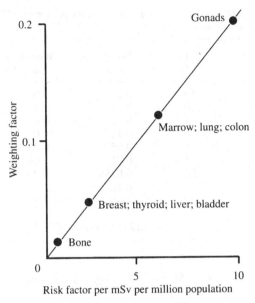

Fig. 4.3. The method of ascribing a weighting factor, used in the calculation of effective dose, for each organ based on the risk of death of an individual after exposure of that organ to radiation.

organs may be irradiated to a different extent. This is taken into account by assigning a weight of 0.05 to the remaining organs without specifically defined weights.

Examples of the calculation of effective dose for two procedures are shown below. The first example is a simple chest X-ray (Table 4.1). Measuring the dose to each organ directly is not possible. Instead the dose to the skin is measured, and a percentage of this dose is ascribed to each organ based on measurements made in phantoms. Weighting factors for the standard organs plus three others, the stomach, liver and heart, are used. These factors are combined with the per cent entry skin dose for each organ to give a series of weighted doses, which are in turn summed to give the effective dose. Thus, for a skin dose of 500 μGy, the gonads will receive 2% of this, or 10 μGy. This gonad dose is multiplied by a weighting factor of 0.2 to give a contribution of 2 μSv to the overall effective dose.

Table 4.2, produced in the same way as Table 4.1, shows quantitatively why long screening times should be avoided because of the high doses that may be encountered in fluoroscopy. In general, effective doses for simple examinations are well below the annual dose from the

Table 4.1. *Calculation of effective dose for a typical X-ray examination. Chest X-ray of female patient: skin entry dose = 500 μGy*

Organ	% entry dose	Dose (μGy)	Weighting factor	Weighted dose (μSv)
Gonads	2	10	0.2	2.0
Breast	2	10	0.05	0.5
Bone marrow (red)	1	5	0.12	0.6
Lung	30	150	0.12	18.0
Thyroid	1	5	0.05	0.25
Bone	1	5	0.01	0.05
Heart	10	50	0.025	1.25
Stomach	5	25	0.12	3.0
Liver	10	50	0.05	2.5
			Effective dose = 28 μSv	

Table 4.2. *Calculation of effective dose for a typical X-ray examination. Screening fluoroscopy: skin entry dose = 40 mGy/min*

Organ	% entry dose	Dose rate (mGy/min)	Weighting factor	Weighted dose rate (mSv/min)
Gonads	0.1	0.04	0.20	0.008
Breast	20	8	0.05	0.4
Bone marrow (red)	0.2	0.08	0.12	0.01
Lung	5	2	0.12	0.24
Thyroid	1	0.4	0.05	0.02
Bone	0.5	0.2	0.01	0.002
Heart	10	4	0.05	0.20
Stomach	5	2	0.12	0.24
Liver	2	0.8	0.05	0.04
			Effective dose rate = 1.2 mSv/min	

For cine fluoroscopy at 50 frames/s and a skin dose of about 0.1 mGy/frame the skin dose rate is 300 mGy/min. This is equivalent to an effective dose rate of about 9 mSv/min.

natural background, and those for complex examinations are around the present annual limit for members of the public. Details of these doses are shown in Table 4.3.

When the range of doses resulting from the same X-ray procedure carried out in different hospitals in the UK is examined, some disquieting features emerge. The spread in dose delivered is shown in Figs. 4.1

Table 4.3. *Effective dose delivered by ten routine X-ray examinations (NRPB, 1986)*

Examination		Effective dose (mSv)	
Category	Type	Median	Range
Simple	Lumbar spine	1.8	0.4 –7.4
	Chest	0.02	0.01–1.3
	Skull	0.15	0.01–0.50
	Abdomen	0.98	0.12–9.9
	Thoracic spine	0.70	0.16–4.4
	Pelvis	1.0	0.09–5.8
Complex	Intravenous urography	3.5	1.4–35.1
	Barium meal	3.0	0.6–24.4
	Barium enema	6.9	2.9–33.6
	Cholecystography	0.6	0.1– 5.0

and 4.2 for examinations carried out in 20 hospitals chosen at random. For each of the examinations a mean value can be calculated, and this may be considered to represent a reasonably achievable guideline dose. The Figures suggest that in some hospitals it appears necessary to give between *three and five times* the guideline dose to achieve acceptable results. This indicates that some equipment in regular use was either faulty or that insufficient care was being taken in quality assurance. Certainly the cardinal principle of 'as low as reasonably achievable' was being ignored in many of these cases. Even wider variations are seen when the comparison is made for the same examination carried out in 'adequate' X-ray departments in different countries, for which variations of 20 to 100-fold can be found.

Factors affecting the dose

The X-ray dose measured at the patient and calculated for each organ is affected by a large number of factors associated with the generation and detection of the X-rays and with the characteristics of the patients themselves (Fig. 4.4). These factors include:

1 *X-ray tube material.* The anode material is chosen to match the beam energy required.
2 *Voltage.* As the voltage increases, patient skin dose and image contrast decrease.
3 *Current.* Higher doses result from higher currents.

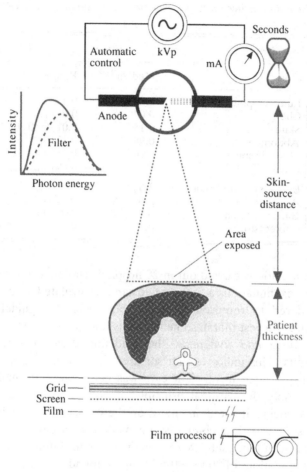

Fig. 4.4. A large number of factors associated with the generation and detection of X-rays and with the characteristics of the patient affect the X-ray dose to the patient.

4 *Time.* The radiation dose delivered is directly proportional to the time of exposure.

5 *Filter material.* Filtration may reduce the skin dose, though it will not necessarily reduce organ doses.

6 *Patient–detector distance.* This should be minimised to reduce the dose.

7 *Area to be imaged.* This should be as small as practicable, consistent with covering the area being investigated.

8 *Patient thickness.* Both scatter and dose increase with patient thickness.

9 *Couch material.* This should have low attenuation to maximise the number of X-rays reaching the film cassette.

10 *Grid.* A grid reduces scatter and improves image quality, but at the expense of increased radiation.

11 *Screen/film combination.* Intensifying screens reduce X-ray dose to the patient.

12 *Film processor.* Under and over-exposure may both lead to examinations and doses being repeated.

The choice of X-ray tube material, voltage, current and time, and the nature and thickness of the filter all contribute in different ways to the dose and thus all can potentially be altered to produce adequate results with a minimum dose. The source–skin distance, area to be imaged and patient thickness may be more difficult to alter. However, the couch material and the use of a grid, the particular screen/film combination and the film processor conditions are suitable elements for optimising quality and reducing dose.

The quality of the image on which the diagnostic value of the examination depends (and thus the whole point of doing the examination) is very much related to the dose. In general, in order to achieve a higher quality image a higher dose has to be incurred by the patient. The image quality depends on a number of features of the object examined and the image itself. These include the instrumental features outlined above and other features of the image such as contrast, resolution and noise.

The dose may be measured at the skin either directly by using thermoluminescent dosimeters (Fig. 4.5), or it may be calculated indirectly given the operating conditions. An additional dose contribution from backscatter, termed the backscatter fraction, must also be taken into account, since it is almost impossible to measure internal doses. There are two methods of calculating the organ dose. These are to use tables of *percentage depth dose* (Fig. 4.6(*a*)) or to use values of *correction factors*, the tissue/air ratios being obtained from measurements in a range of phantoms (Fig. 4.6(*b*)).

Methods of measuring dose

Radiation doses can be measured directly and accurately even in relatively small regions with the use of, for example, thermoluminescent chip dosimeters (Fig. 4.7). Unfortunately the technique is practical only for superficial dosimetry, unless it is performed invasively by

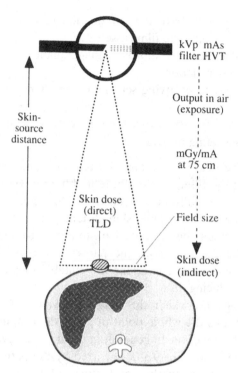

Fig. 4.5. Direct measurement of radiation dose to the skin can be made using a thermoluminescent dosimeter (TLD). It can also be calculated from knowledge of the operating conditions.

inserting the chips, using catheters, into the patient. None the less, a good estimate of gonadal dose can be made by TLD dosimeters fixed to the testicles. Generally speaking, however, the only way of obtaining doses to organs such as the lungs or kidneys is to measure the external dose and then to use either physical or mathematical models to estimate the internal dose.

The process thus involves measuring the skin dose to the patient and applying a correction for the passage of the radiation through the body. Skin doses may be measured either directly with a TLD dosimeter on the skin or by noting various parameters of the X-ray beam (usually with an ionisation chamber device, as illustrated in Fig. 4.8) and reading a dose figure from appropriate tables. From the skin dose and various characteristics of the X-ray beam, the percentage depth dose read from tables gives the organ dose.

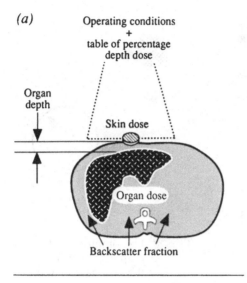

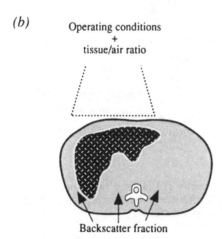

Fig. 4.6. Indirect methods of calculating organ dose depend on (*a*) the skin dose and percent depth dose data or (*b*) use of tissue/air ratio correction factors.

The dose to a particular organ will be determined by the X-ray characteristics, the percentage depth dose, the backscatter fraction (BSF), or, alternatively, the tissue/air ratio (TAR). The BSF and TAR can be determined from separate experiments. These involve direct measurements, using TLD dosimeters, inside phantoms that mimic the X-ray imaging conditions. Further computer calculations can be per-

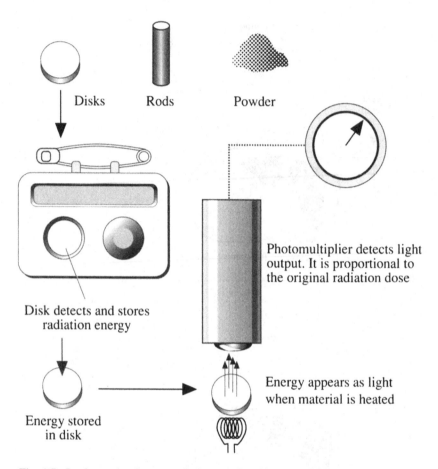

Disks   Rods   Powder

Photomultiplier detects light
output. It is proportional to
the original radiation dose

Disk detects and stores
radiation energy

Energy appears as light
when material is heated

Energy stored
in disk

Fig. 4.7. In thermoluminescent dosimetry (TLD), the radiation dose received
by the dosimeter can be inferred afterwards by heating the material and
measuring the light output using a photomultiplier.

formed to assess scattering and other effects: these involve tracing the
histories of millions of simulated photons through tissue in what is
known as a Monte Carlo simulation.

Radiation doses in nuclear medicine

For radionuclide administration, the radiation dose received by the
organ of interest depends on the effective half-life of the radionuclide
in the organ (a combination of the physical and biological half-lives),
the activity accumulated in it, the absorption factor for each emission

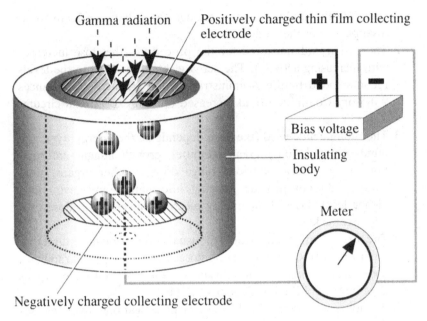

Fig. 4.8. In an ionisation chamber, the positive and negative ions formed by irradiation are separated by an applied electric field. The charges can be collected by conducting electrodes and the radiation dose inferred from the measured current.

from the radionuclide and the geometry of the organ. The total radiation dose to the patient may be due to contributions from a number of organs depending on the metabolic pathways followed by the particular tracer that has been administered. The calculations have been simplified by the production of tables, the 'MIRD' tables (Snyder *et al.*, 1975). These tables enable the dose to be read off for any of the commonly used radionuclides from a knowledge of the activity and time of residence in each organ simulated by standard models of man, of woman, and of children of various ages.

Factors affecting the radiation dose from nuclear medicine procedures

The factors that affect the radiation dose to the patient in nuclear medicine procedures include:

1 The physical half-life of the radionuclide (the dose increases with increasing half-life). The half-life should be long enough to

complete the study, but short enough for radiation effectively to disappear after the study.

2 The activity administered for the procedure (the dose increases with increasing activity). The activity should be kept to the levels recommended by the Administration of Radioactive Substances Advisory Committee (and increased only in exceptional circumstances).

3 The radionuclide used (the dose depends on the energy, type and number of emissions). Gamma emitters provide imaging information but give local and long range dose to other organs. Beta emitters do not provide imaging information and give much higher local doses. Low energy electrons give a high dose at a microscopic level.

4 The organs affected. Although usually one organ is targeted, other organs receive a radiation dose. Tables giving the radiation doses from commonly used isotopes for representative organs have been published by Snyder *et al.* (1975).

5 Physiological factors. In the case of investigations involving isotopes of iodine, for example, the radiation dose to the thyroid may be decreased by blocking it with stable iodine. In general, the radiation dose will be reduced if there is fast excretion.

All the above factors explain why ^{99m}Tc is used so commonly in nuclear medicine. Its half-life of six hours allows tests to be carried out efficiently within a few hours of administration, while the subsequent decay ensures that negligible activity remains after a couple of days. The activity administered may, therefore, be relatively high to ensure good statistical accuracy from the test, and can be increased to allow the test to be completed in a shorter time if the measurement is difficult, as in the case of a small child or a demented patient. The gamma emissions from ^{99m}Tc are at 140 keV, an energy such that attenuation by tissue is not a problem (as it is below about 80 keV) yet one that allows imaging with good efficiency by a gamma camera (which becomes inefficient at energies above about 400 keV). Radiation doses from beta and low energy electron emissions are minimal. In contrast to ^{99m}Tc, the use of ^{131}I involves an isotope with an eight day half-life, gamma energies of over 360 keV, and the presence of beta radiation that contributes about 90% of the total radiation dose, but effectively nothing to the diagnostic information. Table 4.4 lists some of the radiation doses for typical nuclear medicine procedures when activities recommended by the Administration of Radioactive

Table 4.4. *Absorbed radiation doses for typical examinations*

Examination	Effective dose[a] (mSv/examination)	Guideline dose[b] (mGy entrance dose/exam)	
'Simple' X-ray			
Lumbar	2.4	AP 10,	LAT 30
Chest	0.05	PA 0.3,	LAT 1.5
Skull	0.11	AP 5,	LAT 3
Abdomen	1.4	AP 10	
Thoracic spine	0.9	AP 7,	LAT 20
Pelvis	1.8	AP 10	
'Complex' X-ray			
IVU	4.2		
Barium meal	3.4		
Barium enema	7.9		
Cholecystography	0.9		
CT (head and body)	1.1	30	
Nuclear Medicine[c]			
^{99m}Tc bone	5		
^{99m}Tc liver	1		
^{99m}Tc brain	7		
^{99m}Tc lung perfusion	1		
^{99m}Tc kidney (DTPA)	3		

[a] Effective dose represents overall dose (and risk) to body.
[b] Recommended measured surface dose based on NRPB hospital survey.
[c] Doses based on ARSAC recommended administrations.

Substances Advisory Committee are used. The reader is advised to consult the guidance notes issued by this Committee for further information.

Dose reduction also depends on the adequate matching of well-maintained equipment to the imaging conditions. Poor quality images lead to higher patient doses because of the need for higher activities and the possible need to repeat administrations. Matching is achieved through the intelligent choice of collimators and the part of the energy spectrum used.

Summary

X-ray examinations

Table 4.4 shows that there are large variations in the patient dose (effective dose) for different X-ray examinations. This is to be expected, since different organs of different radiosensitivities are involved. However, there are also large variations for the same procedure between hospitals and between countries. This reflects the use of different equipment and, to some extent, different techniques, but also the poor use of equipment (either through default or through misplaced priorities), lack of QA and a basic misunderstanding of quality versus dose and a failure to adopt dose saving measures.

Nuclear medicine

The factors that determine the radiation dose to the patient in nuclear medicine have been calculated and recommendations published by the Administration of Radioactive Substances Advisory Committee (ARSAC). Optimum imaging results using the recommended levels of activity will be obtained only with intelligent use of equipment and regular quality assurance procedures.

References

NRPB (1986). *A National Survey of Doses to Patients Undergoing a Selection of Routine X-ray Examinations in English Hospitals.* NRPB-R200. London: HMSO.

Shrimpton, P. C., Wall, B. F., Jones, D. G., Fisher, E. S., Hillier, M. C., Kendall, G. M. & Harrison, R. M. (1986). Doses to patients from routine diagnostic X-ray examinations in England. *British Journal of Radiology*, **59**, 749–58.

Snyder, W. S., Ford, M. R., Warner, G. G. & Watson S. B. (1975). *"S", absorbed dose per unit cumulated activity for selected radionuclides and organs.* Medical Internal Radiation Dose Committe Report No. 11. New York: Society of Nuclear Medicine.

Wall, B. F., Hillier, M. C., Kendall, G. M. & Shields, R. A. (1985). Nuclear medicine activity in the United Kingdom. *British Journal of Radiology*, **58**, 125–30.

5

The principles of quality assurance and quality control applied to both equipment and techniques

M. WEST

Quality assurance (QA) is a management technique that can be used to moderate any system that results in a product (Hendra, 1986). When setting up a QA programme, it is therefore necessary to define both the final product and the system that produces it. Quality control (QC) comprises the regular testing that must be carried out on each major component of the system to ensure its optimum performance within the system as a whole.

Diagnostic radiology

In the context of diagnostic radiology, QA should be carried out to ensure the production of a high quality diagnostic image for the minimum radiation dose to the patient (NRPB, 1988). QA entails a QC programme that will involve the selective testing of each major system component on a regular basis to ensure its optimum performance within the system (HPA, 1979; BIR, 1988). QA can also include non-equipment matters such as those relating to radiological practice: these are beginning to be matters of public concern (Consumers' Association, 1991).

Systems under quality control

In diagnostic radiology, the major systems to which quality control can be applied are:

1 X-ray production – X-ray tubes and generators.
2 X-ray detection – film/screen combinations and image intensifiers.

3 Image processing – film processors and CCTV systems.
4 Image viewing – film viewers and TV monitors.

These tests must be combined with the routine monitoring of final image quality.

There are many potential tests of X-ray systems, but the most efficient QA programmes are those in which the patient dose reduction is balanced against the cost of staff time, materials and equipment.

X-ray production

Quality control variables for X-ray production include:

1 Tube voltage.
2 Tube current.
3 Exposure time.
4 Automatic exposure devices (AED).
5 Beam filtration.
6 Focal spot size.
7 Radiographic output.
8 X-ray beam/light beam alignment.

All the above should be examined initially to establish a baseline for the QA programme. Regular testing could then be confined to AEDs, radiographic output and, perhaps, beam alignment. However, it could be argued that beam alignment is automatically checked on each occasion that a carefully collimated radiograph is acquired. Weekly measurements should be made on AED devices, especially those used on image intensifier/closed circuit television (CCTV) systems. Some AED devices have a tendency to lose calibration over a period of time and this will affect both image quality and patient dose.

Radiographic output i.e. the radiation dose measured at a fixed distance from the X-ray source for a standard set of exposure factors, is a good indicator of changes in the three major parameters (voltage, current and time). Radiographic output should also be measured on a weekly basis using an ionisation chamber.

X-ray detection

Two types of detector are in common use: film cassettes and image intensifiers.

Film cassettes

Assuming that the most radiosensitive film/fluorescent screen system compatible with the X-ray unit and the required image resolution is already in use, there are three main factors to be considered:

1 Light tightness of cassettes.
2 Uniformity of contact between film and screen.
3 Uniformity of screen sensitivity.

Initially, all cassettes should be tested. Provided a routine visual inspection and cleaning regime is carried out, further QC testing may not be required. All cassettes and screens should be marked so that they can be individually identified from the final radiograph. After initial baseline checks, routine analysis of undiagnostic, or inferior, radiographs should enable simple identification and elimination of sub-standard cassettes.

Image intensifiers

Image intensifiers and their associated CCTV circuits are most easily tested by non-invasive, subjective assessment using standard test objects placed in the X-ray beam and close to the entrance plane of the image intensifier. Such tests are designed to assess the performance of the imaging system from the final image. Typical system tests include:

1 Video signal waveform.
2 Grey-scale linearity.
3 Limiting resolution.
4 Low contrast sensitivity.
5 Uniformity of focus.
6 Geometric distortion.

Once a baseline has been established, weekly or monthly measurements of grey-scale linearity, limiting resolution and low contrast sensitivity should be made, using subjective test objects such as those produced by the Medical Physics Department at Leeds University (Fig. 5.1).

Image processing

Monitoring of film processor efficiency is vital. There is no point in producing the ideal latent image on a film if it cannot be converted to a

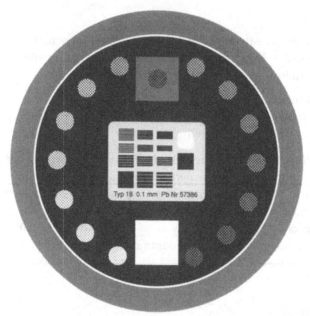

Fig. 5.1. One of a range of test objects for the assessment of X-ray imaging systems produced by the Department of Medical Physics at Leeds.

high quality visual image. *Inefficient processing will increase the radiation dose to every patient examined.*

Most modern processors automatically monitor and control the major parameters such as chemical levels, replenishment and developer temperature but these control systems can be defeated by faults in the system – often simple faults such as blocked pipes. Routine daily monitoring is therefore essential: a reduction of, say, 2°C in developing temperature in the processor may lead to an increase of 20% in patient dose by way of compensation.

The best method of testing processors is to produce a latent image of a grey scale on a film by use of a stable, calibrated, light source (sensitometer: see Fig. 5.2). After processing, the density of the film is measured and the levels of density used to determine:

1 The base fog of the film (i.e. background density).
2 The speed (sensitivity) of the system.
3 The contrast of the system.

These variables should be plotted on a chart to show daily trends and enable operational limits to be set on the performance of the processor (Fig. 5.3).

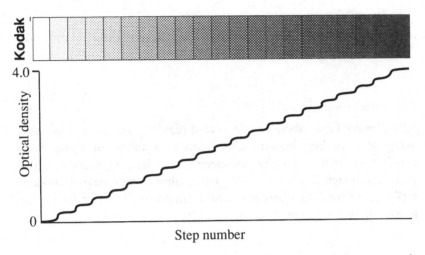

Fig. 5.2. A grey-scale image produced by a sensitometer and the measured film densities.

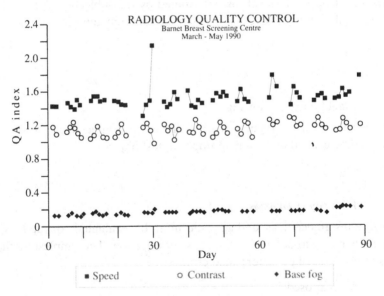

Fig. 5.3. Quality control chart. The steep increase in film speed on day 30 was caused by a blocked pipe in the film processor.

Image viewing

Image viewing conditions are often overlooked, even in the most QA-conscious departments.

Film viewers

Film viewing boxes should be inspected regularly for uniform intensity and colour of illumination. Old fluorescent tubes, or those badly matched in terms of emission spectra, will lead to a reduction in perceived image contrast and may cause films to be repeated unnecessarily. Ambient light levels must also be maintained at a uniformly low level to preserve image contrast.

TV monitors

Contrast and brightness controls should be checked to ensure that they are set at optimum levels as determined by the subjective test objects. Low ambient light levels are essential for high quality TV monitor images.

Final image monitoring

Image intensifiers: regular weekly or monthly subjective assessments should be carried out using appropriate test objects.

Film reject analysis

All films rejected as undiagnostic must be evaluated, on at least a weekly basis, to determine the cause of rejection. The simplest method is to use a set of predetermined criteria:

> overexposed
> underexposed
> incorrect patient position
> movement blurring
> film processing fault etc.

This is known as a reject analysis. An example is shown in Table 5.1.

Table 5.1. *An example reject analysis*

Room	% Rejects due to				
	Under-exposure	Over-exposure	Incorrect position	Patient movement	Film processing
1	25	23	33	13	2
2	27	21	28	15	3
3	20	24	37	10	3
4	19	61	11	6	1
5	22	28	31	11	2

Total number of films used: 2920
Number of rejected films: 372
Reject rate: 12.7%

Major causes, such as individual equipment faults (see Room 4, 'Overexposure' in Table 5.1), can then be identified and eradicated.

Reject rates, which may be as high as 15% of all films taken can, *and should*, be reduced to 5–8%.

Repeated radiographs are the major source of unnecessary patient radiation dose.

Quality assurance related to nuclear medicine procedures

Without QA of the measuring equipment, information from a nuclear medicine procedure may be so poor that an excessive quantity of radioactivity has to be used or the test has to be repeated in its entirety. In practice, significant doses to the patient arise from diagnostic imaging procedures involving a gamma camera and dose calibrator as the main items of equipment, or from therapeutic doses involving a dose calibrator.

QA of dose calibrators is achieved through the regular use of standards that have been calibrated by a national calibration service. These standards are used to check that the equipment is reading within the required limits of, usually, plus or minus about 10%. The results of the checks are recorded so that trends indicating a failing instrument can be identified and appropriate action taken. It should also be noted that such records are required by law, in order, amongst other things, to trace errors in cases of suspected overdosage.

Although rather complex schemes of QA and QC for gamma cameras have been proposed, most of the essential information about the state of the equipment may be obtained by quite simple means, usually involving a check of the uniformity of the camera. This critical check tests the general state of the equipment and yields clues about changes in linearity, the functioning of the photomultiplier tubes and the energy analysis system as well as the uniformity of response. It should be carried out at least once a week by exposing the camera to uniform irradiation from a point source (without the collimator fitted) or a commercially available 'flood' source (with the collimator) of ^{99m}Tc or a long lived analogue such as ^{57}Co. Fig. 5.4 shows an example of such a check. Other tests of linearity, resolution and sensitivity require rather specialised equipment and advice from a centre with a large medical physics department might have to be sought before these are embarked on. Fortunately, once checked on delivery of the equipment, these particular aspects of performance are unlikely to change radically unless modifications are made to the camera.

QC of techniques stems from adequate training of those using the imaging, counting and calibration equipment. The procedures should be established after consultation between doctors, physicists and technicians, written down and followed carefully by all concerned. The procedures include the various settings of the equipment and the positioning of the patient appropriate to each of the tests. Local Rules

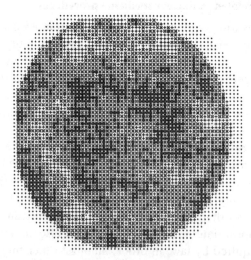

Fig. 5.4. Gamma camera uniformity check: exposure to a flood source.

issued by the radiation protection service must be complied with in order to reduce radiation doses to staff and patients. These will be based on the *Guidance Notes* (NRPB, 1988) and provide information on what to do in the case of accidents and emergencies, checking of activities before administration, segregating patients with high doses, disposal of waste activity etc.

Summary

QA is a management technique that, in diagnostic radiology, should be carried out to ensure the production of high quality diagnostic images for the minimum patient radiation dose. It will require a quality control programme involving the selective testing of each major system component on a regular basis. The major systems in diagnostic radiology concern X-ray production, X-ray detection, image processing and image viewing. For a given system, there are many possible variables that might be monitored, and it is important to balance the potential dose savings against the cost of monitoring. In the case of X-ray production, for example, it may be adequate to confine regular testing to AEDs, radiographic output and beam alignment, once the initial checks have been performed. A QA programme should also include a film reject analysis.

In nuclear medicine, the QA programme should include checks on the dose calibrator as well as checks on the gamma cameras used for imaging.

References

BIR (1988). *Assurance of Quality in the Diagnostic X-ray Department*. London: British Institute of Radiology.

Consumers' Association (1991). X-rays. *Which?* **34**, 40–41.

Hendra, I. R. F. (1986). A systematic approach to quality assurance in medical diagnostic imaging. In *Quality Assurance in Medical Imaging*, pp. 1–14. Bristol: Institute of Physics.

HPA (1979). *Quality Assurance Measurements in Diagnostic Radiology*. CR-29. London: Hospital Physicists' Association.

NRPB (1988). *Guidance Notes for the Protection of Persons against Ionising Radiations Arising from Medical and Dental Use*. London: HMSO.

6

The principles of dose limitation and the various means of dose reduction to the patient, including protection of the gonads

M. WEST

Basic principles

The basic principles of radiation dose limitation are that:

1 All unnecessary doses must be avoided.
2 All necessary exposures should be justifiable in terms of the benefits to the individual that would not otherwise have been received.
3 All doses administered must be the minimum consistent with the medical benefit to the individual.

The most effective way of reducing patient radiation dose is to avoid the use of ionising radiation altogether. For this reason, other methods of obtaining the required information, such as ultrasound or MRI, should be used whenever possible. Every effort must also be made to obtain existing information on the patient in advance, using sources such as records, reports and previous X-rays. The results from recent examinations may contain all the relevant information and preclude the need for further radiation exposure.

Patient dose reduction

If the only acceptable method of obtaining the information required involves the use of ionising radiation, all practical methods of minimising the dose to the patient must be utilised. In diagnostic radiology, the patient dose depends on:

1 The method of obtaining the image.
2 The choice of equipment.
3 The operator's technique.

Methods of obtaining the image

Plain X-ray films should be used in preference to fluoroscopic imaging (screening). Unless *all* the information can be obtained in a total time of about 15 seconds, screening will always incur a higher patient dose. A plain abdominal X-ray, for example, results in a skin dose of about 9 mGy. In contrast, screening is likely to produce dose rates of 30 mGy per minute or more.

Choice of equipment

The correct choice of equipment can considerably reduce patient dose. The following components are especially influential:

1 The X-ray film/fluorescent screen (cassette) combination.
2 The materials used to construct patient support tables, cassettes and antiscatter grids.
3 The X-ray generator type.
4 The filtration of the X-ray beam.

Paradoxically, X-ray film is much more sensitive to light than it is to X-rays. Hence, in the production of a radiograph, the X-rays are made to stimulate light emission from fluorescent screens in the cassette surrounding the film. The efficiency of these screens in converting X-ray energy into light energy, and the response of the film to this light, determine the X-ray dose required to produce an image. Modern, high efficiency systems employing rare-earth phosphors in the screens can reduce the patient dose by a factor of two or more, compared to conventional film/screen combinations.

Any material placed between the patient and the image recording system will increase the patient dose. Some such material, for example the patient support table, will always be present. The increase in dose caused by these materials depends on the percentage of the useful (that is image-forming) X-ray beam that they absorb. Carbon fibre is particularly efficient at transmitting radiation at diagnostic X-ray energies and should be used to replace traditional materials, which may absorb up to 20% more of the X-ray beam.

A diagnostic X-ray tube emits a continuous spectrum of X-ray energies, ranging from a few keV up to the selected tube voltage. X-rays from the lower end of the spectrum do not have sufficient energy to reach the imaging device, but are absorbed in the patient, so increasing the dose without contributing to the diagnostic image.

The precise distribution of energies in the X-ray spectrum depends on the design of the X-ray generator and in particular the manner in which the X-ray tube voltage is produced. Modern generators in which the tube voltage is produced at kilohertz frequencies – the so-called 'medium frequency' or 'multi-pulse' units – produce a high proportion of image-forming radiation and therefore lead to a reduced patient dose.

The X-ray spectrum emitted by a diagnostic X-ray tube is always 'tailored' to reduce the non-image-forming radiation by passing the beam through metal filters that remove the low energy X-rays (Fig. 6.1). Traditionally, beams of energy up to 150 kV have been filtered by a minimum of 2.5 mm of aluminium. Recent work suggests that more selective filtration, using such materials as yttrium and erbium, or heavier filtration with up to 6 mm of aluminium, can reduce the patient skin dose by 50%. However, there is some evidence to suggest that the reduction, in terms of equivalent dose, is considerably less, perhaps as little as 5% (Shrimpton et al., 1988).

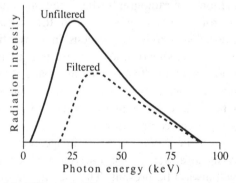

Fig. 6.1. Effect of filtration on the energy spectrum of an X-ray beam: filtration removes the low energy X-rays, which would otherwise be absorbed in the patient without contributing to image formation.

Operator's technique

Individual patient doses may vary considerably, depending on the operator's practical technique. In particular, the following points should be considered:

1 X-ray tube voltage.
2 X-ray beam collimation.
3 Patient–detector distance.
4 Focus–patient distance.
5 Shielding of radiosensitive organs.
6 Choice of projection.
7 Choice of imaging device.

X-ray tube voltage

In general, as X-ray tube voltage increases, patient skin dose decreases, but there will also be a gradual loss of contrast in the final image, which eventually will impair diagnosis. It is therefore important to select the highest tube voltage consistent with an acceptable image quality. The simplest way to ensure this on a fluoroscopy unit is to have the X-ray set fitted with a fully automatic exposure control which will select the most appropriate factors. For conventional X-rays, voltages of 60–120 kV are normally used, with at least 2.5 mm of aluminium filtration. By contrast, in mammography much lower voltages are employed, 28 kV for example, with reduced filtration in order to maximise differential absorption in soft tissue.

X-ray beam collimation

Patient dose depends both on direct irradiation by the main X-ray beam and on secondary, or scattered, radiation that is generated internally. Both the direct and scattered radiation dose can therefore be limited by collimating the X-ray beam so that only the minimum area of the patient is irradiated. Any scattered radiation reaching the detector will degrade the image, since it is not directly related to patient structure. An antiscatter grid placed between the patient and the imaging system will improve image quality but will also increase patient dose, since it will absorb a proportion of the image-forming radiation. Such a grid should therefore be removed, if possible, before examination of children and small adults, from whom the scatter contribution at the detector will be small.

Patient–detector distance

X-ray intensity decreases in air as the square of the distance travelled. If the distance between the patient and the imaging device is increased, there will therefore be a substantial fall in image quality unless other conditions are altered. In particular, a much higher radiation dose will be required if image quality is to be maintained. Wherever possible, therefore, the patient should be kept in close contact with the front surface of the detector.

Focus–patient distance

The distance from the patient to the focal spot should be as large as possible to reduce beam divergence and to minimise entrance dose. *Minimum* focus–skin distances are 30 cm for mobile X-ray sets, 45 cm for stationary equipment and at least 60 cm for chest X-rays.

Shielding of radiosensitive organs

Particularly radiosensitive organs, such as the eyes and the gonads, should be kept out of the direct X-ray beam. Where this is not possible, they should be protected with radio-opaque shields, containing materials such as lead, to the extent that the imaging requirements will allow. In males, for example, the dose to the testes can be reduced by 95% by using gonad shields; in females, the ovary dose can be reduced by 50%. Use of eye shields can reduce eye dose by 50–75%.

Choice of projection

The correct choice of projection can have a considerable influence on the radiation doses received. For example, a PA skull examination will reduce the dose to the eyes by as much as 95% compared with the AP projection; a PA chest X-ray in females will reduce the breast dose by about 95% compared to the AP projection. This substantially reduces the risk of carcinogenesis, so that the AP examination should be carried out only in exceptional circumstances.

Choice of imaging device

Plain X-ray films should be used in preference to fluoroscopic imaging (screening). As already stated, unless *all* the information can be obtained in a total time of about 15 seconds, screening will always incur a higher patient dose. In addition, fluoroscopy poses a potential radiation hazard to the staff. If fluoroscopy must be used, there are a number of imaging techniques available and each will have a bearing on the radiation dose:

1 Pulsed fluoroscopy.
2 Automatic dose rate selection.
3 Magnification (zoom).
4 Image stores and copiers.
5 Video tape recording.
6 100/105 mm cameras.

Pulsed fluoroscopy

It is not necessary for patients to be irradiated continuously during fluoroscopy. The radiation should either be pulsed manually, whenever an image is required, or pulsed automatically.

Automatic dose rate selection

Most modern fluoroscopy units allow a choice of radiation dose rates. The lowest dose rate should always be used as the standard and higher values selected only if this is necessary to improve an otherwise unacceptable image. In general, moving to a higher dose rate will approximately double the patient dose. It should also be remembered that a fluoroscopic image is best viewed in subdued light. High ambient light levels will degrade the image and may lead to the temptation of increasing the radiation dose in order to improve image quality. To obtain high quality TV images in operating theatres, it may be necessary for the surgeon to operate with the aid of a spotlight so that the TV monitor can be viewed under optimum lighting conditions.

Magnification

Magnification of the live fluoroscopic image (zoom technique) is achieved only at the expense of an increased radiation dose – often at double the standard dose rate – and should therefore be used with discretion.

Image stores and copiers

Single TV images from fluoroscopy can be stored electronically and displayed on the TV monitor for review without further irradiation of

Table 6.1. *Typical patient radiation doses in fluoroscopy*

	Relative dose rate	Cumulative skin dose rate (mSv/min)
Minimum dose rate conditions	1	30
Poor collimation	1.3	40 (30 × 1.3)
Increased distance between patient and image intensifier	1.6	60 (40 × 1.6)
'High' dose rate selected	1.6	100 (60 × 1.6)
Magnified image (zoom)	1.6	160 (100 × 1.6)

the patient. Some systems can store multiple images for comparison of, say, AP and lateral views. The potential reduction of the dose by viewing stored, rather than 'live' images, is extremely high. Thermal printers can be used to produce paper copies of these images, which, although of reduced image quality, are usually adequate for the purposes of a record in the patient's case notes and are achieved at a dose below that of a normal X-ray film.

Video tape recording

Unless very high quality dynamic recordings are required, video tape recording should always be used instead of film-based systems such as cine cameras, since the patient dose will be reduced by a factor of about five.

100/105 mm cameras

If high quality, static images are required to be recorded during fluoroscopy, small format (100 or 105 mm) films should be used in preference to standard, large format, radiographs. This will result in a relative reduction in the dose by a factor of between five and ten.

The possible effects of operator technique on patient dose can be seen in Table 6.1. A combination of poor techniques can increase the fluoroscopic dose rate by more than a factor of five.

Summary

It is important to carry out only those X-ray examinations that will produce new information (see NRPB, 1990). The use of alternative imaging techniques should therefore be considered first. If X-rays are employed, then the equipment used must deliver the minimum radiation dose consistent with obtaining the information required. The dose to the patient depends not only on the choice of equipment, but also on the method of obtaining the image and on the operator's technique.

References

NRPB (1990). Patient Dose Reduction in Diagnostic Radiology. *Documents of the NRPB*. Vol. 1, No. 3. London: HMSO.

Shrimpton, P. C., Jones, D. G. & Wall, B. F. (1988). The influence of tube filtration and potential on patient dose during x-ray examinations. *Physics in Medicine and Biology*, **33**, 1205–12.

7

The specific requirements of women who are, or who may be, pregnant and the requirements of children

M. J. MYERS

Introduction

It would be natural to assume that introducing irradiation into the complicated process of cell development in the human fetus would produce some disruption. Popular images of the birth of monsters can be discounted because the self regulatory nature of the development process tends to favour an all or nothing effect (i.e. a normal birth or a termination of the process). Special precautions are, however, called for in dealing with a pregnant, or potentially pregnant, patient. This is because of both the increased risk of radiation damage to the developing fetus and the uncertainties in the clinical situation presented (whether the patient is or is not pregnant calls for quite different strategies of examination).

The child, also, has to be considered as a different radiological proposition from an adult because of differences in body weight, organ size and development that could lead, in general, to overexposure to radiation.

The ten-day rule

From 1970, when the International Commission on Radiological Protection (ICRP) recommendations appeared, until comparatively recently, the main concession to protecting the fetus was the 'ten-day rule'. This rule has had a chequered career (Russell, 1986) and it might, therefore, be appropriate to state the arguments for and against a ten-day rule or, indeed, any other rule related to the menstrual cycle.

The rule (as interpreted by most X-ray and nuclear medicine

departments) recommended that women of childbearing age should be exposed to irradiation involving the pelvis or lower abdomen only during the first ten days after the start of a normal menstrual period. At this time it is reasonably certain that she cannot be pregnant and therefore that there is no risk to a conceptus. The rule was waived if the examination could be properly justified on the basis of health detriment. Certain nuclear medicine procedures such as ^{131}I treatment of thyroid disease were excluded entirely if there was a chance of pregnancy. However, a consideration of the physiological process of the initial phase of development indicates that the risk to a child, who has been irradiated in utero during the remainder of a four-week period after the menstrual period, is small (Fig. 7.1). In fact, the most important period from the point of view of radiation protection is 8–15 weeks (Fig. 7.2).

Considering the need for a diagnostic test for the mother, the risk to the mother of waiting for the next period, according to the old ten-day rule, would be greater than the danger to the fetus. This is especially true if conception was found to have occurred, in which case the test should not be carried out at all. These were the considerations behind the 1984 ICRP revision of the rule which now involves no special limitation on exposure in the four weeks following menstruation.

Also in 1984 the NRPB made the following recommendations:

1 That a woman who has had a missed or overdue period or if, in

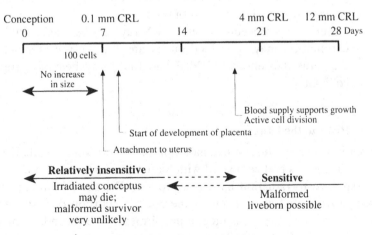

Fig. 7.1. During the first week or two of development of the human embryo it is relatively insensitive to irradiation. CRL, crown–rump length.

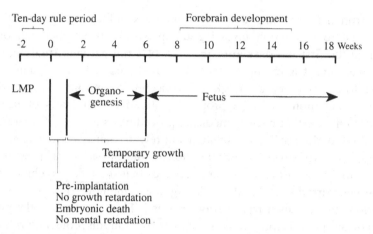

Fig. 7.2. During the first few months of fetal development, the most critical stage from the point of view of radiation protection is the period at 8 to 15 weeks, when forebrain development is occurring. LMP, last menstrual period.

response to the question 'are you, or might you be, pregnant?' cannot answer definitely not, be treated as though she were pregnant. The question must be asked properly and a notice at reception is not sufficient, since language or reading difficulties might lead to its being ignored.

2 If a fetus is known to exist, then efforts have to be made to minimise the number of exposures and the dose from any exposure that directly irradiated the fetus, as long as the diagnostic value of the test is not compromised.

3 Other X-ray procedures, such as X-rays of the chest, skull and extremities, may be carried out at any time in the pregnancy if the fetus if properly shielded and the X-ray beam is properly collimated.

Risks to the fetus

What is at risk because of irradiation *in utero* and what are the risks in numerical terms and compared with 'natural' risks? Two consequences of exposure to radiation have been found. The first, from studies of women irradiated as a means of therapeutic abortion or surviving an atomic bomb explosion, is mental impairment. The second, from very large-scale studies of children with and without fatal cancer (the Oxford Survey of Childhood Cancer), is the incidence of such cancers.

Table 7.1. *Risks of mental retardation*

Weeks post-conception	Probability of radiation related abnormality (/mGy)
0–8	0
8–15	4 in 10 000
16–25	1 in 10 000
> 25	0

Both consequences are extremely hard to detect and to ascribe firmly to diagnostic radiation (rather than, for example in the case of mental impairment, to factors such as malnutrition). The risk factors involved are consequently the subject of some discussion. It is generally agreed, however, that no significant risk of mental retardation exists outside the period at 8–25 weeks post-conception and that the critical period is 8–15 weeks post-conception, when the forebrain is forming (Table 7.1). The risk of mental retardation may be as high as 1 in 2500 per mGy, above a possible threshold of about 250 mGy; however, a linear relationship between the extent of impairment and dose may also fit the experimental data.

The excess risk of cancer is 1 in 40 000 per mGy for the first ten years of life, according to the report of the United Nations Scientific Committee on the Effects of Atomic Radiation (UNSCEAR), and 1 in 5000 per mGy according to the estimates of the Oxford Survey group. The latter group also found a cancer risk after first trimester irradiation that was three times greater than the risk for other prenatal X-rays and six times greater than the risk for children not irradiated in utero. Although the risks seem large, they should be viewed in the context of the absolute number of children with leukaemia and solid tumours. For singleton births, this is of the order of 75 and 50 per 100 000 (with wide ranges of error) in the irradiated and non-irradiated children respectively. There is also a probability of 1 in 30 that a normal pregnancy results in a child with some degree of general handicap and a probability of 1 in 20 that normal pregnancies result in a child with some degree of congenital defect. Nevertheless, the dose to the fetus should be minimised and ARSAC recommends an upper limit of 0.5 mGy unless there is particular justification for exceeding this. The ICRP in 1984 recommended that a pregnancy should be allowed to proceed if the embryo were exposed to less than 100 mGy. Consideration of abortion after accidental fetal irradiation would be justified only at levels very much higher than these, especially since there is a relatively high risk from factors other than irradiation.

With these considerations in mind, there should be a clear local policy for dealing with women of childbearing age presenting in either an X-ray or a nuclear medicine department. A scheme illustrating the process is shown in Fig. 7.3. Dose reduction should also take into account the different body build of infants and children, so that specific X-ray conditions are set for each stage of development.

The 1990 ICRP recommendations in dealing with female workers who are pregnant call for a dose limit to the surface of the women's abdomen of 2 mSv and a radionuclide intake of 1/20 of the annual limit on intake (ICRP 60, 1991). The annual limit on intake, ALI, for each radionuclide is the maximum activity that may be ingested in a year such that a lifetime dose limit of 20 mSv is not exceeded. This limit applies from the time of declaration to the remainder of the pregnancy, and is broadly comparable with that provided for members of the public.

Dose reduction for children in radiology and nuclear medicine

Application of good work practices in the X-ray imaging of children should lead, in general, to much reduced doses. Table 7.2 lists examples of the range of bone marrow doses for common examinations in children of various ages and in adults.

Special X-ray techniques for children include attention to immobilisation (to avoid repeat exposures), shielding, collimation and coning. Added beam filtration generally reduces the proportion of low energy X-rays, which contribute more to dose than to image quality. High speed film/screen combinations however, which in general lead to lower doses, may not, in the case of children, give acceptably high resolution/low noise images and such combinations have to be chosen carefully.

For nuclear medicine, the activity administered to children may be reduced according to a number of schemes. One simple scheme is based on an activity in proportion to the weight of the child with respect to a 70 kg adult e.g. a 10 kg child would require 1/7 of the adult activity. This approximation ignores the disproportionate development of specific organs (such as the brain, which in a one-year-old child is 70% of the adult brain weight). Although this method gives low doses, the practicalities of imaging non-sedated infants, for example, usually

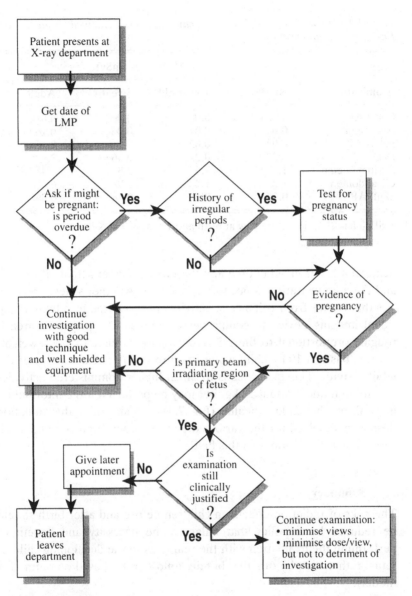

Fig. 7.3. A scheme for dealing with patients who may be pregnant presenting for X-ray examinations. The aim is to minimise the risk of irradiating a fetus. (Adapted from Wilks, 1987).

Table 7.2. *Mean dose estimates to active marrow. Adapted from Hilton, Edwards & Hilton (1984)*

Examination	Mean dose (mSv)			
	Newborn	1-year-old	5-year-old	Adult
Chest AP	0.004	0.005	0.008	0.014
Abdomen AP	0.04	0.04	0.06	0.16
Pelvis AP	0.02	0.02	0.1	0.16
IVU	0.27	0.27	0.46	2.1
Barium enema	1.3	1.6	2.3	7.4
CT abdomen	1.2	1.4	1.9	6.4
Skull AP[a]	0.15	0.14	0.18	0.06

[a] Skull has 27% active marrow at birth and 7% at 40 years.

demand a faster imaging time and therefore a higher activity if the test and the administration is not to be repeated. Another scheme recognises that counts from volumes of activity are converted by a two-dimensional imaging device to counts per unit area. The projected area is roughly proportional to the 2/3 power of the volume or body weight. On this basis, a 10 kg child would require $(1/7)^{2/3}$ or about 1/4 of the adult activity. This factor leads to much higher administered activities for children under about 10 kg, but may be preferred if the information is vital to the child's health (Fig. 7.4). In all cases the radiation dosimetry involved for the various organs is rather imprecise and much work remains to be done in this field.

Summary

The risks of radiation effects on children before and after birth should be reduced by a policy that balances the necessity and benefit of performing the irradiation with the real risks to the developing child or fetus, rather than by one that blindly follows rules based on outmoded models.

There should be clear local policies on:

1 Avoiding the irradiation of a pregnant or potentially pregnant woman, while still obtaining essential information.
2 Keeping radiation doses to children as low as possible by special X-ray techniques and by reducing radionuclide activities administered.

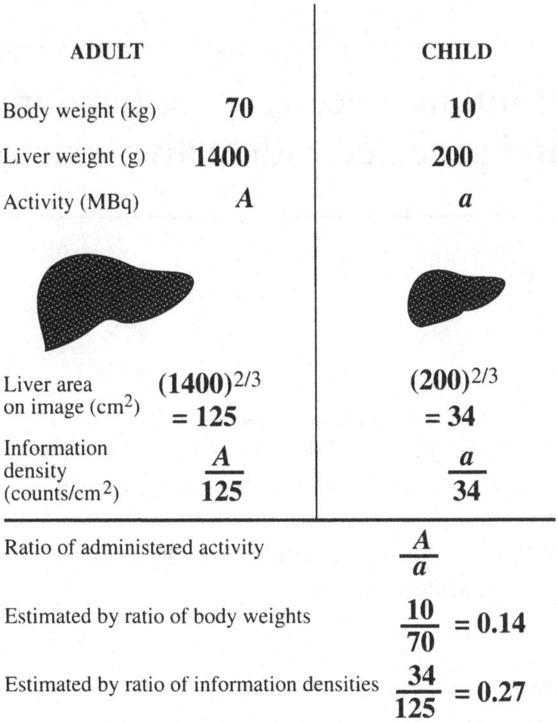

ADULT	CHILD
Body weight (kg) **70**	**10**
Liver weight (g) **1400**	**200**
Activity (MBq) **A**	**a**

Liver area on image (cm^2)	$(1400)^{2/3}$ = 125	$(200)^{2/3}$ = 34
Information density (counts/cm^2)	$\dfrac{A}{125}$	$\dfrac{a}{34}$

Ratio of administered activity $\dfrac{A}{a}$

Estimated by ratio of body weights $\dfrac{10}{70} = 0.14$

Estimated by ratio of information densities $\dfrac{34}{125} = 0.27$

Fig. 7.4. Two schemes for calculating the activities to be administered to a child from those for an adult. One method is to reduce the activity in proportion to the child's bodyweight. A better scheme may be to use the two-thirds power of the ratio of the bodyweights, which leads to rather higher activities being administered.

References

Hilton, S. W., Edwards, D. K. & Hilton, J. W. (1984). *Practical Pediatric Radiology*. Philadelphia: Saunders.

ICRP 60 (1991). *1990 Recommendations of the International Commission on Radiological Protection*. ICRP Publication 60. Oxford: Pergamon Press.

Russell, J. G. B. (1986). The rise and fall of the ten-day rule. *British Journal of Radiology*, **59**, 3–6.

Wilks, R. J. (1987). *Principles of Radiological Physics*. Edinburgh: Churchill Livingstone.

8

The precautions necessary for handling sealed and unsealed radioactive sources

K . C . K A M

The emphasis of this chapter is on the reduction of doses to staff who handle sources of radioactive materials, rather than the reduction of doses to patients who receive high doses in the course of their therapy with these materials.

Radioactive sources in clinical use can be broadly divided into two categories: sealed and unsealed sources.

Sealed sources

The radioactive material in a sealed source is usually in powder or solid form and is encapsulated in a casing made from a metal such as platinum or stainless steel. In normal use there is, therefore, very little danger of spreading the radioactivity through contamination; the hazard comes mainly from the radiation emitted from the source.

Most sealed sources are used for the purposes of radiotherapy. Examples include ^{137}Cs needles and tubes, ^{198}Au grains, ^{192}Ir wires and ^{90}Sr beta ray ophthalmic applicators. Fig. 8.1 shows the appearance of a variety of sealed sources for clinical use. Many are reusable with working lives of up to ten years. There must, therefore, be a source storeroom in which the sources are kept when not in use. This is a legal requirement in the UK and in most other countries. The room should be equipped with a safe for the storage of the sources and a workbench with sufficient shielding for their preparation and cleaning. A suitable meter should be available to monitor the radiation dose rate in the vicinity. A set of Local Rules (example A; see p. 81), a system of work, contingency plans for dealing with accidents (example B; see p. 82) and a map showing the storage location of each source must be clearly displayed in the room. Further information is contained in the

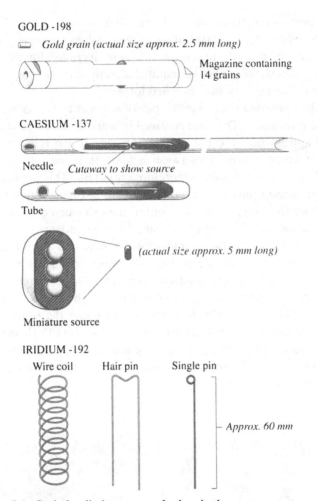

GOLD -198

Gold grain (actual size approx. 2.5 mm long)

Magazine containing
14 grains

CAESIUM -137

Needle   Cutaway to show source

Tube

(actual size approx. 5 mm long)

Miniature source

IRIDIUM -192

Wire coil   Hair pin   Single pin

Approx. 60 mm

Fig. 8.1. Sealed radiation sources for brachytherapy.

Approved Code of Practice (HSC, 1985) and the *Guidance Notes* (NRPB, 1988).

Members of staff who have to handle the sources or who have to nurse or examine patients in whom the sources have been inserted or implanted must try to minimise the radiation exposure to themselves. The three ways to minimise personnel exposure when handling sealed sources are by using distance, speed and shielding:

 1 *Distance*. The distance between sources and personnel should be maximised. The dose rate falls off rapidly as the square of the

distance from a radiation source. If the distance is doubled, the dose rate reduces to a quarter of its original value; conversely if the distance is halved, the dose rate will increase fourfold. Hence, sources should never be handled directly with the fingers, but always with a pair of long-handled forceps.

2 *Speed*. The operating time spent by personnel near to the sources should be minimised. The dose received in working with a source is directly proportional to the time of exposure to the radiation. That is, if an operation takes twice as long, then the radiation dose will be doubled. Speed is therefore important. This requires good organisation and preparation. It means getting everything ready before the sources are taken out of their shielded container for preparation, for cleaning or for using them on patients.

3 *Shielding*. Shielding between radiation sources and personnel should be employed when possible. The most commonly used materials for shielding are lead and concrete. Fig. 8.2 shows a typical radiation source storage bench unit. At the back of the bench are lead storage safes with drawers to house the sources. At the front of the bench is a lead brick wall 4–5 cm thick with lead glass observation windows for the protection of the operator when manipulating the sources. Sources are transported using a lead trolley (Fig. 8.3).

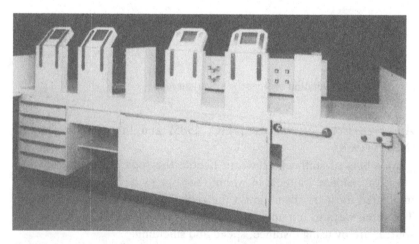

Fig. 8.2. A typical radiation source storage bench unit. There are lead shields and lead glass observation windows in front of the bench and lead safes with individual drawers at the back.

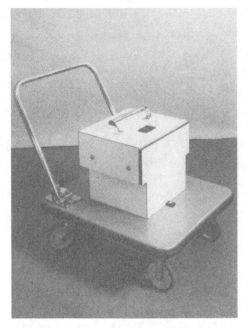

Fig. 8.3. A lead trolley for the transportation of radiation sources within a hospital.

To ensure the protection of members of staff who have to nurse or examine patients who have been inserted or implanted with radioactive material, a mobile bed shield of lead 3–4 cm thick is usually employed (Fig. 8.4).

All sealed sources have to be accounted for before, during and after each use. Reusable sources, such as ^{137}Cs, have to be cleaned up after each use and returned to the safe for storage afterwards. Other sources have to be stored in a separate safe for radioactive decay and then returned to the suppliers for disposal.

All the swabs, dressings and linen used in the insertion or implant procedure must be checked with a radiation monitor to ensure that they are free from contamination before they can be disposed of. This is especially important in the case of ^{198}Au grain implants. The sources are so tiny that one or two grains may come loose from the implant and lodge in the patient's dressings. After the removal of the sources, the patient should also be monitored to ensure that no source has been left behind.

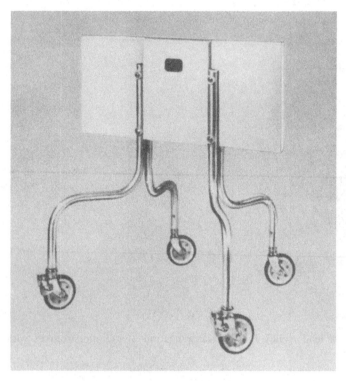

Fig. 8.4. A mobile, lead bed shield for placing between the nursing staff and the bed to reduce the radiation dose to personnel.

Unsealed sources

Most unsealed sources are radionuclides used for diagnosis, treatment or research. They are usually supplied in liquid or colloidal form in a variety of containers (Fig. 8.5). Examples of unsealed sources include ^{99m}Tc, ^{131}I, ^{32}P, ^{51}Cr and ^{59}Fe. They are administered to patients by injection, by mouth or used for in vitro tests. When handling unsealed radioactive substances, a radiation hazard may arise either through external irradiation of the body by the source or through the entry of a radioactive substance into the body by ingestion or by inhalation. Unsealed sources may produce a further external radiation hazard as a result of environmental contamination.

The main precautions required in dealing with external irradiation are similar for both sealed sources and unsealed substances i.e. the use of distance, speed and shielding. Most of the unsealed substances used

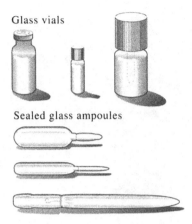

Fig. 8.5. Containers for unsealed radionuclides.

for diagnostic purposes are of low activity and therefore the amount of shielding required can be reduced accordingly.

However, additional measures are required to prevent the spread of radiation hazard through contamination. Laboratories and other working areas used for the manipulation of unsealed sources should have smooth and non-absorbent surfaces for the room, benches, tables and seats, so that they can be cleaned and decontaminated easily. Members of staff should wear protective clothing and waterproof gloves. All manipulations should be carried out over a drip tray (Fig. 8.6) lined with absorbent paper in order to minimise the spread of contamination due to breakages or spills.

All contaminated pipettes, syringes and bottles with residual sources should be sealed in labelled plastic bags for storage and subsequent disposal through the waste disposal service. All other materials and apparatus used in a procedure should be monitored for contamination before they can be disposed of or put away.

No food or drink, cosmetics or smoking materials should be brought into a laboratory, and paper tissues should be used instead of handkerchiefs.

High activity patients in a ward

Patients who have been given a therapy dose of an unsealed radionuclide, e.g. ^{131}I, should be confined to a single room with its own toilet and washing facilities. The room should incorporate adequate radiation

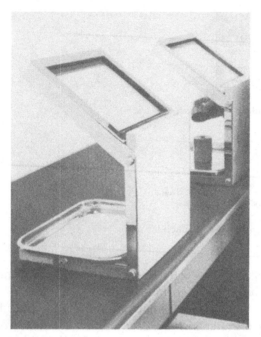

Fig. 8.6. A stainless steel drip tray behind an L-shaped lead shield.

shielding and should be a side room in a general ward away from the staff and the general public. The floor of the room should be covered with absorbent paper to contain the spread of contamination from urine, faeces, vomit etc.

Disposable crockery and cutlery should be used, and should be collected with any left over food in a plastic bag for monitoring before being disposed of. If such items are contaminated, they should be treated as radioactive waste for the purposes of disposal.

Nursing and other procedures that are not urgent should be postponed for as long as possible. Patients should be encouraged to do as much for themselves as practicable. Protective gowns and gloves should be worn when excreta, contaminated clothing, bed linen or other articles are handled.

Summary

All radioactive sources, both sealed and unsealed, are potentially hazardous if they are not handled properly. The precautions to be taken in order to reduce exposure to personnel are, however, simple and, in many instances, based on common sense. The three basic principles of: (1) maximising distance; (2) minimising handling time; and (3) using protective shielding, are by far the most effective ways to reduce radiation dose. In general, they can all be applied at the same time. However, there are occasions when only one or two of these principles can be employed. For example, it is inconvenient to use shielding when a radiotherapist has to implant radioactive iridium hairpins into the tongue of a patient. In this case, speed and good preparation prior to the operation are the most important factors. Members of staff who have to handle radiation sources should have prior knowledge of the type and the activity of the sources they are going to deal with so that the appropriate precautions can be taken. The Ionising Radiations Regulations 1985 require each establishment working with ionising radiations to have a set of Local Rules and written systems of work for each type of work involving radiation in order to minimise radiation exposure to staff. It is the duty of each employee to familiarise themselves with these rules and procedures and put them into practice.

Example (A)   Sealed radiation sources store room: Local Rules

1.   Introduction

The store room is located on the ground floor by the south side of the South Corridor near D-Block. It is a purpose-built room providing radiation protection all round. It houses two main safes and two supplementary safes. Each has its own specific contents:

  (a) Radiotherapy safe – containing all pre-loaded ^{137}Cs sources in the form of uterine tubes and ovoids.
  (b) Physics safe – containing all discrete sources of ^{137}Cs, ^{226}Ra, ^{241}Am, ^{198}Au and ^{192}Ir.
  (c) Green caesium safe – containing all pre-loaded ^{137}Cs line sources.
  (d) Iridium bin – containing all used iridium wires and hairpins.

2.   Designation of Areas and Limitation of Access

The store room is a permanent CONTROLLED AREA, and a warning sign is displayed on the door. Entry of non-classified staff must be in accordance with a written System of Work.

3.   System of Work

  3.1 Film badges must be worn at shoulder level when manipulating sources on the bench.
  3.2 All sources must be handled with long forceps or the mechanical hand behind the lead wall, preferably by looking through the mirror.

3.3 Do not stand in front of the bench unnecessarily while sources are being sterilised or being soaked to be cleaned.

3.4 Take out from the safe only the sources that are required.

3.5 All sources should be put back in the appropriate safe as soon as they have been cleaned.

3.6 No sources should be left unshielded on the bench overnight.

3.7 The door should always be locked if the room is unattended.

3.8 No sources may be taken out of the room unless they are in a suitable protective container.

3.9 Issue or return of sources must be recorded in the appropriate book.

3.10 The contents of each safe must be checked periodically and recorded.

3.11 The Iridium Bin should be emptied regularly of used wires. All wires are to be returned to Amersham for disposal.

Example (B)   Actions to be taken in the event of suspected or known loss of a sealed source: Local Rules

Sealed solid sources are either stored, prepared or in use in the following locations within the hospital site:

1. Operating Theatre.
2. Radioactive Sources Store Room.
3. Hot Laboratory – Department of Medical Physics, basement of Commonwealth Building.
4. Radiotherapy Department – Physics Laboratory (1st floor) and Treatment Rooms (basement), Supervoltage Building.
5. Wards I5 and 6 – 2nd floor, I Block.
6. Radiodiagnostic Department – 1st floor, J Block.

The radiation sources commonly in use are:

1. Caesium-137 (tubes and miniature sources).
2. Cobalt-60 (tubes and cylinders).
3. Gold-198 (grains).
4. Iridium-192 (pins and wires).
5. Radium-226 (tubes and needles).
6. Strontium-90 (ophthalmic applicators and calibration standards).

In the event of known or suspected loss of a radiation source:

1. The person who discovers the loss must inform, without delay, the Radiation Protection Supervisor (RPS) of the relevant department, or the person in charge at that time.
2. The RPS or the person in charge must, in turn, inform a physicist at whatever hour of day or night (see list of emergency telephone numbers) and work should proceed under his or her direction.
3. The Radiation Protection Adviser should also be informed.
4. Before the arrival of the protection physicist, there should be no sweeping of floors, no disturbing of equipment, furniture, sinks, sluices or

toilets, no movement or disposal of soiled dressings, laundry or dustbins, and minimal movement of staff or patients.

5. The search for the lost source should be carried out by the physicist using a suitable instrument, assisted by the RPS, using methods appropriate to the circumstances.

   a) If a source is lost from a patient or near a patient, and there are other sources in use inside or on the patient, all the removable items used by and in the vicinity of the patient should be monitored one by one in a low radiation background area. The patient should then be moved with the bed or trolley to a place known to be free of radioactivity and away from other patients and staff. The original area should then be searched and monitored.

   b) If it is suspected that a source has been lost from a patient in transit e.g. from operating theatre to wards or to the radiology department, the search should then be extended to cover the entire route along which the patient has been transported.

   c) If it is suspected that a source has been lost in the laboratory during preparation (e.g. cutting and loading of ^{192}Ir wires, loading ^{137}Cs miniature sources onto moulds or applicators), it may be difficult to locate the strayed source with a survey monitor due to the high radiation background from other sources in storage in the vicinity. In this case the known sources should be loaded into a protective container and transferred to other parts of the laboratory before proceeding with the search. Special attention should be paid to the possibility that the lost source might have fallen into a gap between protective materials.

6. If all the above actions to recover the lost source have failed, the search should then be extended to cover the refuse reaching the incinerator, bed-linen etc. in the laundry and drains from the sluices or toilets. If necessary, assistance should be summoned either from the National Radiological Protection Board or through the National Arrangements for dealing with Incidents involving Radioactivity (NAIR).

7. Should there be any reason to suspect that the lost source might have become damaged, the possibility of contamination by spilled radioactive substances should be borne in mind. At the earliest indication of such contamination, appropriate precautionary measures should be instituted at once.

References

HSC (1985). *Approved Code of Practice. The Protection of Persons against Ionising Radiation Arising from any Work Activity.* London: HMSO.

The Ionising Radiations Regulations 1985. Statutory Instrument No. 1333. London: HMSO.

NRPB (1988). *Guidance Notes for the Protection of Persons against Ionising Radiations Arising from Medical and Dental Use.* London: HMSO.

9

Organisation for radiation protection.
The organisational arrangements for
advice on radiation protection and how
to deal with a suspected case of
overexposure

A. BRADLEY

Organisation

The use of ionising radiation in the diagnosis and treatment of patients
is covered by various regulations in the UK. The Ionising Radiations
Regulations 1985 and 1988, the Radioactive Substances Acts 1948 and
1960 and the Medicines (Administration of Radioactive Substances)
Regulations 1978 all cover aspects of this work. Broadly speaking, this
legislation, together with the Health and Safety at Work Act, is
designed to place the onus on health authorities to ensure the safety of
staff, patients and members of the public while they are on their
premises and to ensure their safety from discharges of radioactivity
into the environment. The majority of hospitals employ a large number
of staff, in a wide variety of departments, many of whom will be
exposed to radiation during the course of their work. It is therefore
essential that a health authority has a suitable administrative organisation in place to ensure that the work is carried out safely and that none
of the various regulations is contravened.

This chapter deals with the type of organisation suitable for hospitals and the responsibilities of the various members of staff involved. It
is based on the information contained in the *Guidance Notes for the
Protection of Persons Against Ionising Radiations Arising from Medical
and Dental Use* (NRPB, 1988). An example of the administrative
organisation suitable for a hospital is shown in Fig. 9.1.

The Health and Safety at Work Act puts the responsibility for safety

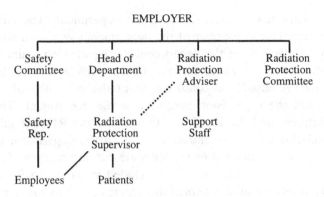

Fig. 9.1. Administrative organisation for radiological safety. An example from the *Guidance Notes* (NRPB, 1988).

on the *employer*. This will probably be the appropriate health authority. However all *employees* have a duty to ensure that anything they do endangers neither themselves nor anyone else. The Ionising Radiations Regulations require health authorities to appoint a Radiation Protection Adviser (RPA) to advise on all aspects of radiological safety. The Radiation Protection Adviser should be a physicist with experience in radiation physics, who has an understanding of the work being undertaken in the establishment concerned.

The Health and Safety Executive must be informed of, and acknowledge, the appointment of an RPA. The RPA will usually be a member of the hospital staff but could also be a member of an outside organisation engaged to provide RPA services to the hospital. If the range of hazards is diverse, more than one RPA may be appointed e.g. one covering radiotherapy and another for diagnostic radiology.

The RPA should assess the hazards present in a department and draw up any necessary schemes for the safe conduct of work. Regular visits should then be made to ensure that the schemes are effective and to review them where necessary. The regulations require that employers provide the RPA with the information and means necessary for the fulfilment of this task.

Health authorities will usually delegate responsibility for a department to the head of that department, who will then be responsible for the radiation safety of the staff and any patients or visitors in that area. The head of department should, therefore, be involved in drawing up safety measures in consultation with the RPA.

A Radiation Protection Supervisor (RPS) must be appointed to supervise the work that is carried out in the department. The RPS should be an experienced member of the department's own staff who will normally be available in the department during working hours; a consultant who works elsewhere for part of the week would not be suitable. The RPA should be consulted about the suitability of an appointment and the supervision necessary in the department. The head of department and the RPS, with the help of the RPA, should draw up Local Rules for the conduct of work in the department to ensure that the schemes devised by the RPA are put into practice. The name of the RPS responsible should be included in the Local Rules and should be known to all members of the department. Any problems they encounter should be reported to the head of department who has the responsibility for seeing that action is taken.

Some hospitals may have a radiation protection committee to aid the process of consultation between RPAs and the departments. The committee should comprise the heads of departments, the RPA and a representative from the hospital administration. If it is feasible, the departmental RPSs should also be involved in the committee.

Record keeping

The regulations insist on good record keeping. Table 9.1 provides a summary of some of the records that have to be kept and the length of time for which they must be kept.

Other records that should be kept are details of diagnostic examinations both to patients and to volunteers, radiotherapy treatments, the administration and removal of radioactive implants and the daily movements of radioactive sources. For a more exhaustive list, see the *Guidance Notes* (NRPB, 1988).

Controlled and supervised areas

If the level of radiation in an area is such that an employee who works in the area could receive a radiation dose that exceeds 3/10 of any statutory dose limit, either the whole body dose limit or an extremity dose limit, then the regulations require the area to be designated a controlled area. An area should also be designated as a controlled area if there is a major hazard from radioactive contamination. Entry to a

Table 9.1. *Records and the length of time for which they must be kept*

Record	Number of years
Personnel radiation dose records	50
Radiation dose assessment following an accident	50
Results of an overexposure investigation	50
Investigation of losses of radioactive substances	50
Monitoring of controlled and supervised areas	2
Disposal of radioactive waste	As specified by the DoE

controlled area must be restricted to classified radiation workers or other persons working to a written system of work. The area must be physically demarcated, and the entrance marked with a warning notice, which incorporates a radiation warning symbol (Fig. 9.2(*a*)). It is common that X-ray rooms are designated as controlled areas only when the generator is connected to the mains power supply. In this situation, the warning signs are often of an illuminated type that are not visible when switched off. They are wired into the generator mains supply so that they are illuminated when the generator is switched on (Fig. 9.2(*b*)). In this case, the Local Rules would specify that the room is a controlled area when the sign is illuminated.

The regulations require that the area should be designated as a supervised area if an employee working in it might exceed 1/10 but not 3/10 of any dose limit, i.e. there is a hazard but it is not as great as that within a controlled area (note that ICRP 60 suggests a different definition for controlled and supervised areas). Access should again be restricted and a sign should indicate the designation of the area and the restrictions in force.

The Local Rules for a department should contain details of all controlled and supervised areas and the restrictions that apply to each.

Classified persons and systems of work

Any person who is likely to exceed 3/10 of any dose limit, whole body or extremity, must be designated as a classified radiation worker and be subject to medical and dosimetric monitoring. It is not likely that any person working in a hospital will need to be designated at present, with the exception of some interventional radiologists or radiopharmacists in busy departments, whose finger dose may approach the

(a)

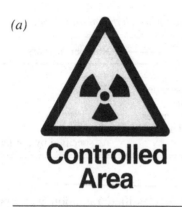

(b)

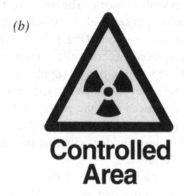

Fig. 9.2. Signs at the entrance to a controlled area: *(a)* is a conventional sign; *(b)* is illuminated. (Both signs comprise black lettering on a yellow background.)

extremity limit. This means that a written system of work has to be prepared for everyone who may be required to work in a controlled area, including all radiographers, radiologists, nurses and engineers. These systems of work have to be designed so that if members of staff follow their guidelines the dose they will receive will not exceed the classification limit.

Personal monitoring

Strictly speaking, only classified radiation workers need to have their personal dose assessed by means of a dosimeter. However it is usual to monitor the majority of staff who work with radiation as this is the easiest way of ensuring that the systems of work are effective in keeping radiation doses below the classification level and as low as reasonably achievable. Personnel radiation doses can be assessed using one or more dosimeters, which are worn on the appropriate part of the body. Two main types of dosimeter are used, film badges and thermo-luminescent dosimeters (for further details, see Chapter 4). A dosi-meter should be worn on the trunk between chest and waist height. This allows an assessment of the dose to the whole body to be made. Other dosimeters may be issued to measure the doses to the extremi-ties, eyes or the thyroid. If a lead apron is being worn, the dosimeter should be worn under the garment, as it will then measure the dose that the trunk has received and not the higher dose received by the outside of the lead apron (lead aprons are quite effective at absorbing scattered radiation). Other dosimeters may be worn to measure the dose to exposed organs if the dose these organs are expected to receive is likely to be significant. The length of each monitoring period will depend upon the dose levels expected (usually 4 weeks for film badges and 13 weeks for TLDs). Dosimeters must be returned promptly for assessment at the end of a monitoring period otherwise they lose sensitivity and an accurate assessment of the radiation dose becomes impossible. A record of the doses received by personnel has to be kept for 50 years and should be openly available for an individual to check on their recent or cumulative exposure. Formal investigations have to take place if a non-classified employee's dose exceeds 3/10 of any dose limit. However, local informal investigations involving the RPA and relevant RPS would usually be instigated if a monthly dose exceeded 1/10 of any limit.

Overexposure incidents

In the event of an accident resulting in an employee or patient being exposed to radiation, an investigation has to be carried out by the RPA to ascertain the causes and to estimate the dose received by the person(s) involved. A report may have to be sent to the Health and Safety Executive (HSE) if the radiation dose to a member of staff exceeds the legal limit, and the HSE may also follow up with its own investigation. To help with this process, all relevant details should be noted down at the time of the incident. In the case of accidents with X-ray equipment, the generator setting (voltage, current etc.) and the position of the person(s) at the time of the incident should be included, at the very least. If radioisotopes were involved, then the isotope, activity, radiopharmaceutical (if appropriate) and details of what happened are required. If the radiation dose to a member of staff is thought to be of concern, such as the accidental exposure of a pregnant member of staff, then their personal dosimeter can be sent for immediate processing to give a better assessment of the dose they received.

Summary

The organisational arrangements for radiation protection in an establishment such as a hospital will involve the appointment of a Radiation Protection Adviser and one or more Radiation Protection Supervisors. These individuals, together with the heads of the departments concerned, will draw up written systems of work and Local Rules to ensure safe practices. This may entail the designation of certain places as controlled or supervised areas.

References

ICRP 60 (1991). *1990 Recommendations of the International Commission on Radiological Protection.* ICRP Publication 60. Oxford: Pergamon Press.
NRPB (1988). *Guidance Notes for the Protection of Persons against Ionising Radiations Arising from Medical and Dental Use.* London: HMSO.

10

Statutory responsibilities

M. J. MYERS

Legislation

In the UK, work with ionising radiation is governed by a number of pieces of legislation, from both the domestic and the European Community Parliaments (Fig. 10.1). Two Acts have formed the basis of the controlling legislation, the Health and Safety at Work Act of 1974, which has led to the Ionising Radiations Regulations 1985, and the European Communities Act 1972, which has led to the Ionising Radiation (POPUMET) Regulations 1988. All the legislation has the aim of creating safe practices such that radiation doses to patients, workers and the general public are kept to a minimum consistent with achieving the required diagnostic or therapeutic result. In particular, the object is to reduce dose levels below deterministic thresholds, thus avoiding deterministic effects, and to minimise the probability of unavoidable stochastic effects.

Since the Regulations are very far reaching, covering a wide range of work from high level nuclear fuel processing to low level radio-immunoassays, they are necessarily rather general and couched in legalistic language. This makes it difficult to apply them directly to everyday hospital situations. A succession of documents seeking to clarify and make practical the Regulations has thus been introduced.

The next level of legislative document after the Regulations themselves is the *Approved Code of Practice* (HSC, 1985). The third level of documentation is the very practical *Guidance Notes* (NRPB, 1988). While the Regulations and the *Code of Practice* have equal standing in the strict sense of the word, the *Guidance Notes* are rather like the Highway Code in having a quasi-legal status. However, it would be difficult to defend unjustified contravention of the *Guidance Notes*.

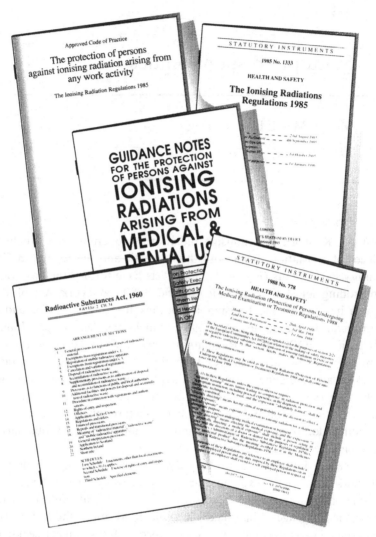

Fig. 10.1. A plethora of legislation.

The keeping, disposal and use of radioactive material is regulated by the Radioactive Substances Act, 1960, which was last revised in 1991. Anyone wishing to use radionuclides of activity above a certain low level must be authorised by the Department of the Environment after having satisfied the Inspectorate about a number of issues including possible hazards to the public. Transfer and transport of radioactive materials is also covered by a number of statutory instruments. The

Radioactive Substances Act and transport regulations would normally be the concern of the Radiation Protection Service of the hospital, rather than the person using or administering the isotope. Administration of radioactive materials to patients (and research subjects) is regulated by the Medicines (Administration of Radioactive Substances) Regulations, 1978, whereby only those holding certificates issued by the Health Minister through the Administration of Radioactive Substances Advisory Committee (ARSAC) may administer or, under special conditions, delegate administration of radioactive substances to persons.

Two bodies make recommendations affecting the way in which the legislation is carried out in practice. These are the International Commission on Radiological Protection (ICRP) and, in the UK, the National Radiological Protection Board (NRPB). It is through the work of these bodies that the dose limits for exposure to radiation are effectively reduced from the legal limits (ICRP 60, 1991). Other reports, among the many available, deal with the *Radiation Dose to Patients from Radiopharmaceuticals* (ICRP 53, 1987), the *Annual Limits on Intake of Radionuclides by Workers* (ICRP 61, 1991), *Protection of the Patient in Radiation Therapy* (ICRP 44, 1985) and *Nuclear Medicine* (ICRP 52, 1987), and *Data for Use in Protection against External Radiation* (ICRP 51, 1987). Reports from the NRPB are also valuable in giving practical guidance. There is, for example, *Organ Doses from Medical X-ray Examinations Calculated Using Monte Carlo Techniques* (NRPB, 1985) and *A National Survey of Doses to Patients Undergoing a Selection of Routine X-ray Examinations in English Hospitals* (NRPB, 1986).

In a similar fashion, the POPUMET Regulations require all persons who 'authorise or effect exposures' to have adequate training in those aspects of radiation protection related to diagnostic or therapeutic work that is not purely scientific research. Further, they must possess proof of this training in the form of a recognised certificate. This proof is required when applying for ARSAC authorisation and by the employing authority, who have a duty to keep records of the training particulars of their staff.

The Ionising Radiations Regulations

The range of subjects covered by the 1985 Ionising Radiations Regulations includes:

1 Dose limitation; restriction of exposure and dose limits.
2 Regulation of work with ionising radiation; controlled areas; organisation of protection service and training.
3 Dosimetry and medical surveillance; aspects of dosimetry services.
4 Arrangements for control of radioactive substances; keeping and transporting radioactive material.
5 Monitoring of ionising radiation.
6 Assessments and notifications; hazard assessment and investigations of (over) exposures.
7 Safety of articles and equipment.

As an example of the legal language used in the Regulations, the section on dose limits for the whole body is reproduced below.

The dose limit for the whole body resulting from exposure to the whole or part of the body, being the sum of the following dose quantities resulting from exposure to ionising radiation, namely the effective dose equivalent from external radiation and the committed effective dose equivalent from that year's intake of radionuclides, shall in any calendar year be —

(a) for employees aged 18 years or over,   50 mSv
(b) for trainees aged under 18 years,   15 mSv
(c) for any other person,   5 mSv

The Approved Code of Practice and the Guidance Notes

The above example is amplified in the *Approved Code of Practice.* However, the language is still rather legalistic and despite its name the *Code of Practice* is not very easy to adapt to practical situations. Thus, for example, the term committed dose is defined as follows:

The words 'committed dose equivalent' refer to the dose equivalent accruing over the period of 50 years following the intake of radioactive material. Once the committed dose or committed effective dose equivalent has been assessed for a particular dosimetric period it is attributed to that period for the purpose of compliance with the dose limits. Thus the only effective method of controlling and limiting the committed dose quantity is by controlling and limiting the intake.

In the *Guidance Notes* (NRPB, 1988), the level of discussion takes on a more practical character. For example, the use of dose equivalent:

For convenience, research projects, should be categorised, according to the level of effective dose equivalent as given in Tables 1 and 2. Only for the most compelling reasons should experiments giving effective dose equivalents greater than those for category III be undertaken. Wherever possible, the effective dose equivalents to normal control subjects should be no greater than those for category II.

Table 1. *Categories of research project involving irradiation of human beings*

	Category		
	I	II	III
Effective dose equivalent	Less than 0.5 mSv	More than 0.5 but less than 5 mSv	More than 5 but less than 50 mSv

etc.

It can be seen from the above that, except as a last resort, advice should be sought in the *Guidance Notes*.

Organisation of responsibilities

Statutory responsibilities are, strictly, more likely to be ascribed to the employer rather than the employee. However, duties are delegated down a chain of appointed persons such as the Radiation Protection Adviser through to the employee who is responsible for his or her own safety and that of others. It is of vital importance, quite literally, that the spirit and intent of the statutory instruments are carried out by those involved in work with ionising radiations. Advice, therefore, on taking note of Local Rules, warning signs, schemes of work in controlled areas, dose monitoring, record keeping and keeping radiation doses as low as reasonably achievable should be followed as if it were legally binding even on those occasions when it is not.

Summary

Work with ionising radiation is strictly controlled by law so that patients, workers and the general public are exposed to the minimum radiation hazard arising from that work. The most practical source of general advice is to be found in the *Guidance Notes* (NRPB, 1988). Because the legislation is constantly being updated in the light of changing knowledge, the local Radiation Protection Adviser should be consulted for more detailed or more up to date information.

References

HSC (1985). *Approved Code of Practice. The Protection of Persons against Ionising Radiation Arising from any Work Activity*. London: HMSO.

ICRP 44 (1985). *Protection of the Patient in Radiation Therapy*. ICRP Publication 44. Oxford: Pergamon Press.

ICRP 51 (1987). *Data for Use in Protection Against External Radiation*. ICRP Publication 51. Oxford: Pergamon Press.

ICRP 52 (1987). *Protection of the Patient in Nuclear Medicine*. ICRP Publication 52. Oxford: Pergamon Press.

ICRP 53 (1987). *Radiation Dose to Patients from Radiopharmaceuticals*. ICRP Publication 53. Oxford: Pergamon Press.

ICRP 60 (1991). *1990 Recommendations of the International Commission on Radiological Protection*. ICRP Publication 60. Oxford: Pergamon Press.

ICRP 61 (1991). *Annual Limits on Intake of Radionuclides by Workers Based on the 1990 Recommendations*. ICRP Publication 61. Oxford: Pergamon Press.

NRPB (1985). *Organ Doses from Medical X-ray Examinations Calculated Using Monte Carlo Techniques*. NRPB-R186. London: HMSO.

NRPB (1986). *A National Survey of Doses to Patients Undergoing a Selection of Routine X-ray Examinations in English Hospitals*. NRPB-R200. London: HMSO.

NRPB (1988). *Guidance Notes for the Protection of Persons Against Ionising Radiations Arising from Medical and Dental Use*. London: HMSO.

11

The choice of diagnostic or therapeutic procedures: clinical value in relation to other techniques

M. RODDIE

Background

As medicine has become more sophisticated, the demand for diagnostic investigations has increased dramatically. Nowhere has this been more evident, or more costly, than in departments of diagnostic radiology, where there has been a 5% increase in work load, year after year since 1966 (Wrighton & Oliver, 1980) resulting in a widening gap between what is technically possible and what is economically feasible. As medical imaging and interventional radiological techniques become more numerous and more complex, it is difficult for even the most motivated non-radiologist to remain fully informed about recent developments. It is, however, non-radiologists who are initiating the majority of investigations and in most centres prior consultation with a radiologist is largely confined to the more complex investigations such as computed tomography, magnetic resonance scanning and angiography. This results in expensive and inefficient use being made of diagnostic facilities.

Reasons for rationalising use of radiography

There are three main reasons for trying to reduce the number of inappropriate investigations being performed. Radiation protection for the patient is the first and most important reason. In the UK, the total effective dose to the population from artificial sources is about 18 000 man Sv (NRPB, 1989) and most of this dose, some 92%, arises from diagnostic X-rays. Age is a critical factor in determining risk, with the fetus and developing child being more radiosensitive than the adult.

Radiation risks may range, for example, from a 1 in 3 million chance of inducing a fatal cancer if an elderly patient has a chest radiograph to a 1 in 140 chance of producing mental retardation if a fetus is exposed inadvertently whilst its mother is having a barium enema examination in the period between 8 and 15 weeks of pregnancy (Kerr, 1991).

Financial considerations must also be taken into account, as the increase in demand for radiological services has not been matched by a corresponding increase in resources. Although doctors are loath to consider management of their patients on a financial basis, it must be recognised that health service budgets are finite.

Limitation of patient investigation by financial constraint imposed from outside the profession is undesirable and the best use of available facilities must be decided by the medical profession itself. Several studies have shown that significant savings can be made by simple changes in practice, without a detrimental effect of patient care. For example, it is known that out-of-hours radiographs do not always influence patient management. Charny *et al.* (1987*b*) estimated that 6 million pounds could be saved by the NHS each year, if the number of radiographs taken was not reduced but instead they were performed during normal working hours.

Finally, if a large number of 'routine' investigations (to exclude rather than to confirm a diagnosis) are performed, large waiting lists build up and the efficiency of the radiology department decreases.

Royal College of Radiologists' Working Party

In 1975, the Royal College of Radiologists established a Working Party with the aim of promoting more effective use of diagnostic radiology. At the first meeting it was stated that 'radiologists are very concerned about the increasingly expensive and often inefficient use that is being made of diagnostic facilities. Correction of the situation would lead to greater efficiency in patient management, reduction in radiation exposure, and reduction in the cost of the service'. It was concluded that the College should produce a series of advisory guidelines to help hospital doctors and general practitioners to make the best use of their local X-ray department. A series of national, multicentre studies were established to answer questions about the effectiveness, safety and cost of five commonly used diagnostic radiological procedures: pre-operative chest radiography, skull radiography in head injury, lumbar spine radiography in the management of back pain, radiography of injured limbs, and abdominal radiography in the management of the acute abdomen. Guidelines based on the results of these studies have been published (Fowkes *et al.*, 1984, 1987; Charny *et al.*, 1987*a*; Hayward *et al.*, 1984) and were summarised in *Clinical Radiology* in 1987 (Fowkes *et al.*, 1987). The College has since issued a useful booklet, which is reproduced in the Appendix, in order to emphasise to the medical profession as a whole the need for conservative use of X-rays (Royal College of Radiologists, 1987). Use of such guidelines can, for example, reduce pre-operative chest radiography by 50% and skull radiography in an Accident and Emergency department by 50%, without any harmful effect on patient care.

Alternative imaging techniques

When there is no alternative to the use of ionising radiation, it is often possible to reduce the number of views performed. The Joint Working Party undertook a limited survey of 62 hospitals and found quite a marked variation in the number of projections used routinely in certain types of examination. It has been shown that instead of performing three separate views of the paranasal sinuses, a single occipito-mental view, with attention to radiographic technique, is sufficient for diagnostic purposes. Others have recommended that a single lumbar spine radiograph is sufficient in the initial investigation of low back pain (Padley *et al.*, 1990) and that if computed tomography (CT) of the back is to be undertaken, then plain radiographs can be omitted altogether in the first instance (Tress & Hare, 1990). Thought should also be given to the type of follow-up examination used. Although a particular examination may be necessary for initial diagnosis, an alternative, less expensive or lower radiation dosage imaging technique may be adequate for follow up. Investigation of vesicoureteric reflux in children is a good example of this principle. The initial diagnosis is made using micturating cystourethrography but adequate follow up can be obtained using radionuclide imaging, which is less invasive and results in a lower radiation dose (Gordon, 1990).

Ultrasonography and magnetic resonance imaging (MRI) do not use ionising radiation and the former has the additional advantage of being a cheap, portable and readily available form of imaging. MRI has replaced CT as the imaging modality of choice for the central nervous system and musculoskeletal system and applications for the chest and abdomen are continually being developed and refined. MR angiography, although still in an early stage of development, may eventually replace conventional angiography. MRI, however, remains expensive and is not available in all hospitals. No significant side effects have been demonstrated with either of these newer techniques and they should be used whenever possible. For example, ultrasonography has replaced oral cholecystography in the investigation of suspected gall stones and should also be used in screening for liver metastases in oncology patients. Although some patients will require CT to clarify ultrasonographic findings, a significant number can be managed adequately using ultrasound alone. Ultrasonography is also the imaging method of choice for both the male and female pelvis, particularly with the advent of rectal and vaginal probes.

The relative use in any given hospital of 'non-radiological' imaging (for example, endoscopy, colonoscopy and arthroscopy) and their conventional radiological counterparts (double contrast barium examinations and arthrography) will depend on local expertise and length of waiting lists. It is preferable, however, to employ the technique that does not use ionising radiation in order to adhere to the ALARA principle, which states that the patient's radiation dose should be as low as reasonably achievable.

Patient dose reduction

A number of measures can be taken in a radiology department to reduce the patient's radiation dose. The use of rare-earth screens and carbon fibre components in the table tops, antiscatter grids and cassettes has been recommended (BIR, 1986). Good technique during fluoroscopy (without a grid where possible) and use of collimation and compression, when appropriate, are also important. If appropriate, radiosensitive organs such as the gonads and eyes should be shielded. It is important to perform regular inspections of apparatus, particularly image intensifiers. Periodic measurement of patient doses should be performed and appropriate action taken if guideline doses are exceeded. Each department should have a quality assurance programme to check the performance of both staff and equipment. One way of analysing staff performance is to perform an analysis of reject films. A group closely aligned to the Working Party has reported on the frequency with which radiographers at different hospitals repeat films (Rogers et al., 1987). The overall repeat rate was 10%, although nearly half of the departments exceeded this and one department repeated almost 20% of all films. The study demonstrated that poor exposure due to errors by the radiographer or the machine accounted for most of the repeats. Expensive devices can be installed for automatic exposure control, but simpler measures such as exposure charts in each room and callipers to measure the size of the patient can be just as effective (Watkinson *et al.*, 1984). In future, the widespread introduction of digital radiography is likely not only to reduce the radiation dose per procedure but virtually to eliminate the incidence of repeat films caused by incorrect exposure factors (Kushner *et al.*, 1986; Kogutt *et al.*, 1988).

Summary

Improved use of a radiology department can be achieved by minimising the number of inappropriate investigations and by good radiographic technique. The former depends upon referring clinicians and guidelines have been issued to help him or her to select the most useful radiological examination in a given clinical circumstance. Patients will be investigated most appropriately, however, in hospitals in which there is a successful and close working relationship between the doctors inside and outside the radiology department.

References

BIR (1986). Low-attenuation materials and rare-earth screens in radiodiagnosis. *British Journal of Radiology*, **59**, 745.

Charny, M. C., Ennis, W. P., Roberts, C. J. & Evans, K. T. (1987*a*). Can the use of radiography of arms and legs in accident and emergency units be made more efficient? *British Medical Journal*, **294**, 291–3.

Charny, M. C., Roberts, G. M. & Roberts, C. J. (1987*b*). Out-of-hours radiology: a suitable case for audit? *British Journal of Radiology*, **60**, 553–6.

Fowkes, F. G. R., Davies, E. R., Evans, K. T., Green, G., Hugh, A. E., Nolan, D. J., Power, A. L., Roberts, C. J. & Roylance, J. (1987). Compliance with the Royal College of Radiologists' guidelines on the use of pre-operative chest radiographs. *Clinical Radiology*, **38**, 45–8.

Fowkes, F. G. R., Evans, R. C., Williams, L. A., Gehlbach, S. H., Cooke, B. R. B. & Roberts, C. J. (1984). Implementation of guidelines for the use of skull radiographs in patients with head injuries. *Lancet*, **ii**, 795–6.

Gordon, I. (1990). Urinary tract infection in paediatrics: the role of diagnostic imaging. *British Journal of Radiology*, **63**, 507–11.

Hayward, M. W. J., Hayward, C., Ennis, W. P. & Roberts, C. J. (1984). A pilot evaluation of radiography of the acute abdomen. *Clinical Radiology*, **35**, 289–91.

Kerr, I. H. (1991). Patient dose reduction in diagnostic radiology. *Clinical Radiology*, **43**, 2–3.

Kogutt, M. S., Jones, J. P. & Perkins, D. D. (1988). Low-dose digital computed radiography in pediatric chest imaging. *American Journal of Roentgenology*, **151**, 775–9.

Kushner, D. C., Yoder, I. C., Cleveland, R. H., Herman, T. E. & Goodsitt, M. M. (1986). Radiation dose reduction during hysterosalpingography: an application of scanning-beam digital radiography. *Radiology*, **161**, 31–3.

NRPB (1989). *Radiation Exposure of the UK Population – 1988 Review*. NRPB-R227. London: HMSO.

Padley, S., Gleeson, F., Chisholm, R. & Baldwin, J. (1990). Assessment of a single lumbar spine radiograph in low back pain. *British Journal of Radiology*, **63**, 535–6.

Rogers, K. D., Matthews, I. P. & Roberts, C. J. (1987). Variation in repeat rates between 18 radiology departments. *British Journal of Radiology*, **60**, 463–8.

Royal College of Radiologists. (1987). *Making the Best Use of a Department of Radiology – Guidelines for Doctors*. London: Royal College of Radiologists.

Tress, B. M. & Hare, W. S. C. (1990). CT of the spine: are plain spine radiographs necessary? *Clinical Radiology*, **41**, 317–20.

Watkinson, S., Moores, B. M. & Hill, S. J. (1984). Reject analysis: its role in quality assurance. *Radiography*, **50**, 189–94.

Wrighton, R. J. & Oliver, R. M. (1980). Trends in radiological practice in the NHS. *Health Trends*, **12**, 21–4.

12

The importance of existing radiological films and reports

M. RODDIE

Introduction

It has been estimated that approximately 20% of radiological examinations requested are inappropriate or unnecessary (NRPB, 1990). Truly inappropriate examinations can be minimised by giving full clinical information on the request form, including details of previous radiological examinations and stating exactly what information it is hoped will be obtained from the examination. In an ideal world, all requests would be checked by a radiologist before being carried out. In practice this is not possible in most departments, but a satisfactory alternative is for clinicians to consult a radiologist for advice about any case where the choice of investigation is not clear cut. A booklet, published by the Royal College of Radiologists, containing guidelines for commonly used examinations, is also available (see Appendix).

Repeat examinations

A significant number of investigations (estimated to be as high as 10% in some hospitals), are unnecessary repeats because the previous study has been lost (NRPB, 1990). Until radiology departments become totally digital and picture archiving and communication systems (PACS) become widely available, the problem of lost or mislaid radiographs will remain. At present, if images are lost, automatic repetition of the study is almost never necessary. There will be a copy of the report, filed in the main radiology department or available from the radiology information system, which may give all the information that is required for patient management. If the study has been lost before reporting, it should be possible to obtain the relevant information by speaking to the radiologist who performed the examination. In certain circumstances, such as the fracture clinic, the report is of less value to the referring clinician than the radiograph itself and there may be no option but to perform a repeat examination. Such occurrences should, however, be kept to minimum. In order to prevent films becoming lost in the first place, radiology departments should have an efficient filing system and prompt or instant reporting of examinations. Clinicians can play an important role by becoming familiar with the way their own radiology department handles and stores radiographs. Some hospitals have found that filing inpatient films in a designated area, with its own viewing facilities in the radiology department, reduces the traffic of films into and out of the department and hence the incidence of lost or mislaid film packets.

Another form of unnecessary repeat examination occurs when a 'gold standard' imaging modality is used to monitor a patient's response to treatment. For example, a mass, initially imaged by computed tomography for full assessment, can usually be followed up perfectly adequately using ultrasonography. Likewise, a plain film follow up of a contrast study may be all that is necessary. Plain abdominal radiographs usually suffice to monitor the progress of a radiopaque calculus, initially demonstrated using intravenous urography.

Previous studies

Finally, a patient's previous radiographs are often of crucial importance in interpreting current studies. The radiological interpretation of a nodule seen on a chest radiograph, for example, is totally dependent on the appearance of previous radiographs. If the nodule was present on the radiograph of five years ago it will be interpreted as a benign lesion, but if it was not present on the radiograph taken six months previously it is likely to be malignant. In the former case, ignorance of the findings of previous studies may, therefore, result in inappropriate and possibly dangerous further investigation for a benign lesion. Similarly, in patients with previous tuberculous disease, detection of reactivated disease or the development of a scar carcinoma will be difficult without old radiographs for comparison. Many studies, such as ultrasonography or renography of transplant kidneys, can be interpreted only by comparison with previous studies and are virtually useless in their absence.

Summary

Attention paid to a patient's previous radiographs and reports will avoid unnecessary repeat examinations. Ignoring or not reading reports leads to patient morbidity and mortality and, with the growing public awareness and anxiety about ionising radiation, to possible litigation.

References

NRPB (1990). Patient Dose Reduction in Diagnostic Radiology. *Documents of the NRPB*. Vol. 1, No. 3. London: HMSO.

13

Priorities for spending in the national health service

B. F. WALL

Introduction

In all countries of the world today the provision of health care is characterised by an insatiable demand and by finite resources. No matter what level of development a country may have achieved, people's expectations for medical services tend to rise in proportion to the resources and technology that are made available, and although priorities may change from country to country, the need to establish priorities for health care spending remains universal.

In the UK, medical radiology, being at the high technology end of the spectrum of health care services, already consumes a large proportion of hospital budgets. Any further investment to nullify unwanted side effects in the form of individually small radiation risks, has to compete with all other patient care services on offer, many of which may appear to represent more cost effective ways of improving the health of patients than does radiation protection. In an ideal world, the allocation of a hospital's or a health authority's resources would be based on the principle of spreading the maximum health benefit equitably among the maximum number of people. Radiation protection suffers from a considerable disadvantage in this competitive environment due to the delayed and intangible nature of the benefits it bestows. Health service managers are frequently unsympathetic to the idea of spending now in order to save later, especially when 'later' could be decades later and the saving, in terms of a few potential delayed deaths, is by no means readily apparent.

A somewhat simplistic but none the less useful method for making comparisons between the cost effectiveness of radiation protection options and other medical procedures is discussed in the next section. An indication that radiation protection can sometimes offer better value for money, it is followed by an outline of some basic decision aiding techniques to help X-ray department staff and hospital managers assess their local priorities and the need for spending on patient dose reduction. The use of such techniques was recommended in a recent report on patient dose reduction in diagnostic radiology prepared jointly by the Royal College of Radiologists and the National Radiological Protection Board (NRPB, 1990). Medical physicists acting as Radiation Protection Advisers play a crucial role in this decision making process by encouraging the development and implementation of appropriate techniques. It should be appreciated, from the outset, that these techniques merely provide an input into what is often a more complex decision. The ICRP publication on *Optimization and Decision-making in Radiological Protection* (ICRP 55, 1989) contains more detailed information on these techniques, which medical physicists might find useful.

Economic appraisal of medical procedures

One simple method of economic appraisal that has been applied to health care programmes is cost effectiveness analysis. It seeks to compare the relative effectiveness of alternative ways of spending health service resources by expressing their outcome in terms of a single common indicator. A particularly useful indicator that has found wide acceptance is the number of years of life gained, together with a measure of the quality of that life. This is expressed as the number of Quality Adjusted Life Years or QALYs. The adjustment for quality of life allows the method to be applied to medical procedures that enhance life as well as those that extend it. It necessarily requires a system for quantifying parameters like pain, anxiety and disability such as the one developed by Kind *et al.* (1982).

If the number of QALYs gained by adopting a particular radiation protection option in diagnostic radiology can be estimated, together with the cost of implementing the measure, then the cost per QALY gained provides a means for comparing the radiation protection option with established medical procedures that have been assessed in the same way. The appropriateness of diverting money away from accepted health care procedures towards improved patient protection can then be judged more properly.

This type of analysis was carried out for patient protection measures involving the use of low attenuation carbon fibre components in X-ray equipment by Wall & Russell (1988). These procedures were chosen because they involve significant expenditure for replacing components and are accompanied by only moderate reductions in patient dose. If these are shown to be relatively 'cost effective', then it follows that other protection measures involving less expense and/or greater dose savings should be given even higher priority. These measures also have the advantage of reducing the dose to the patient without affecting the dose to the image receptor, so that quantum noise in the image will not be increased to the detriment of image quality. If image quality is degraded by the protection measure, this would introduce a further 'cost' into the analysis that would be exceedingly difficult to quantify in monetary terms.

Estimates of QALYs gained from radiation protection measures depend critically on many assumptions regarding, for example, the risk coefficients used for calculating radiation effects per unit dose, the age distribution of patients, the delay between exposure and death, and the quality of life prior to cancer death and for those suffering from non-fatal cancers. The radiation risk coefficients used by Wall & Russell (1988) and the method for predicting years of life lost were essentially those contained in ICRP Publications 26 (ICRP 26, 1977) and 45 (ICRP 45, 1985) respectively. The costs of implementing the protection measure and the total potential dose saving will depend on local conditions such as the anticipated working life of the modified equipment and the patient workload over this period. Assuming a ten-year working life and a patient workload typical of an average general purpose radiography room, Wall & Russell (1988) estimated the costs per QALY gained from various uses of carbon fibre components, as shown in Table 13.1. The table also includes similar estimates for established medical procedures for comparison. All costs are expressed in 1983/4 prices.

These estimates are very approximate and those for radiation protection measures will probably need revising in view of recent changes in the models used to predict the delayed health effects of radiation exposure. However, the necessary revision is likely to be much smaller than is suggested by the threefold increase in the radiation risk coefficients (ICRP 60, 1991). This is because the majority of radiation-induced cancers are now predicted to occur later in life, when they will have less impact on the number of years of life lost. While one awaits these detailed revisions, which will undoubtedly cast radiation protection measures in an even more favourable light, the estimates in Table

Table 13.1. *Costs per QALY for radiation protection measures and medical procedures. From Wall & Russell (1988)*

	Cost per QALY (£)
Radiation protection measures	
Carbon fibre in antiscatter grids	540
Carbon fibre in film cassettes	1800
Carbon fibre table tops	2400
Medical procedures	
Neonatal intensive care	100
Pacemaker implant	700
Hip replacement	750
Heart valve replacement	900
Coronary artery bypass grafting (3 valve disease, moderate angina)	2400
Kidney transplant	3000
Mammographic breast screening	3300
Percutaneous transluminal coronary angioplasty (1 vessel disease, moderate angina)	3400
Cervical screening	3750
Heart transplant	5000
Kidney dialysis (at home)	11 000
Kidney dialysis (in hospital)	14 000

13.1 indicate that even relatively expensive protection options, such as carbon fibre table tops, already compete favourably with a number of medical procedures that consume significant health service funding. This should help to quell the doubts of those who question the wisdom of directing limited health service resources towards radiation protection and away from more visible forms of health care.

Assessing priorities in patient protection

The effectiveness of different methods of patient dose reduction can be compared simply in terms of the expected collective dose saving over the operating lifetime of the proposed method. To be truly indicative of proportionate reductions in collective radiation detriment, the 'collective dose' saved should be a reasonable estimate of the collective *effective dose*. Medical physicists are probably in the best position to assess the potential collective dose savings from a proposed method of dose reduction. It can often be estimated simply from a knowledge of the percentage dose reduction the method is likely to achieve, and the collective effective dose anticipated for the equipment in question over its remaining working life. This will obviously be a function of the types of X-ray examination conducted on the equipment and the patient workload.

If an estimate of the total financial costs of applying each method is also available, those methods that are definitely not cost effective can be immediately rejected. This merely requires that the methods are listed in order of increasing costs and those costing more but not providing a larger collective dose reduction than preceding methods are excluded as not being cost effective. Future costs should be assessed at their present value using standard discounting procedures, or more simply by annualisation.

There are dangers however in comparing the remaining 'cost effective' methods solely in terms of the cost per man Sv saved which, it might be thought, would allow the methods to be arranged in a sensible order of priority. If the intention is merely to select the most suitable single method of dose reduction from a range of alternatives, the appropriate choice will depend on whether the amount of money available for radiation protection is fixed or whether a specific dose reduction is required.

If the intention is to arrange the methods into an order of priority and then apply each one in turn until resources are exhausted, a judgment based solely on the relative costs per man Sv saved of each method applied independently, may also be incorrect. This is because the approach does not allow for the successive diminution of the 'baseline' collective dose after each protection method has been applied.

However, this effect can be allowed for in a form of *incremental* cost effectiveness analysis where all possible combinations of the available protection options are listed in order of increasing costs and then analysed in terms of the incremental costs and dose savings involved in moving from one combination to the next. In essence the most cost effective combination is the one in which the ratio of the *additional* cost to the *additional* benefit is a minimum. Prior to such analysis, those combinations that are definitely not cost effective should be eliminated in the same way as for the individual methods. The incremental cost effectiveness, expressed in £ per man Sv, then determines the order of priority, and indicates how far one can proceed along a series of protection options before the law of diminishing returns seriously compromises the cost effectiveness.

Table 13.2. *Illustrative incremental costs per unit dose saving in a hypothetical radiology department*

Equipment modification	Incremental cost effectiveness (£ per man Sv)
Rare-earth screens	2–20
Carbon fibre grids	50–1500
Carbon fibre cassettes	200–1000
Carbon fibre table tops	250–4100

Illustrative ranges for values of the incremental cost effectiveness have been calculated by Croft (1988) for a number of dose saving modifications to X-ray equipment applied in a hypothetical radiology department and these are listed in Table 13.2. The range of values shown for each equipment modification arises from two sources.

First, there will be a number of different possible combinations for the potential dose saving modifications in each room of the department. The range of values quoted covers all cost effective combinations terminating in the specified option, i.e. it is the spread in *incremental* cost effectiveness achieved by *adding* the specified modification to a number of possible combinations (including zero). The incremental cost effectiveness of the specified modification will diminish as the number of alternatives preceding it increases.

Second, the ranges quoted in Table 13.2 for the same equipment modification cover the values found for different rooms in the department. The costs and the effectiveness can vary considerably because of differences in patient workload and in the remaining working life of the equipment; this indicates the need to base these estimates on local conditions.

Overall, the values range from £2–£4100 per man Sv saved. If they have not already been installed, rare-earth screens are usually found to be the best buy.

In this example, adventitious cost savings that might result from the proposed equipment modification, such as the ability to install a cheaper, lower power X-ray generator or the delayed replacement cost for the X-ray tube, when changing over to faster rare-earth screens, have not been taken into account. In some cases these can result in a long term cost *saving* for the protection measure, in which case the need for its implementation is irrefutable. Health service managers should find this a convincing argument.

Cost effectiveness analysis thus provides a useful way for assessing priorities for spending on radiation protection in the National Health Service. It encourages budget holders at least to make assessments of the doses delivered to patients by their existing radiological procedures, of the potential for reducing doses by alternative methods and of the financial costs of doing so. All of these are necessary components of quality assurance and medical audit, and provide an invaluable aid to hospital managers when deciding how best to deploy any scarce resources that might become available for the purposes of radiation protection.

Comparisons with other industries

A number of studies have been published of investment in safety measures in the nuclear industry and of their effectiveness in reducing collective dose either to workers or to the general public. Fernandes-Russell *et al.* (1988), in summarising such studies, stress that, particularly for major safety systems, investment decisions in the nuclear industry are based on many considerations other than the potential radiation detriment. The costs of serious accidents will be dominated by the costs of the ensuing clean up, of providing alternative power supplies and by political reactions. For this reason, only valuations of the man Sv implicit in investment decisions for reducing doses during normal operations of nuclear plant are shown in Table 13.3. They are taken from Fernandes-Russell *et al.* (1988) and can be compared with the corresponding values for a hypothetical X-ray department shown in Table 13.2. The valuations are expressed in terms of £000s per man Sv at the base year indicated in the Table.

In diagnostic radiology, the cost per man Sv, even for relatively expensive items such as carbon fibre table tops, is on a par with the lowest figure shown in Table 13.3 and nearly three orders of magnitude lower than the highest figure. This enormous disparity serves only to emphasise the very high standards of safety expected of the nuclear industry, and the apparently much greater tolerance of risks that are accepted voluntarily in the context of health care. Although one recognises that investment in safety is ultimately driven by public demand, it is reasonable to question whether the above Tables indicate

Table 13.3. *Valuations of the man Sv implicit in investment decisions in the nuclear industry*

Area of investment	Year	£000/man Sv
Doses to workers		
at Sizewell B PWR[a]	1986	4–160
at French PWRs[a]	1983	7–2000
at CANDU reactors	1986	7–68
at Canadian U mines	1986	1500
in French U mines	1986	20–116
Doses to public		
from USA PWRs[a]	1977	11–3800
from French PWRs[a]	1986	550–1300
from Sellafield	1987	1400

[a] PWR, pressurised water reactor.

excessive spending in the nuclear power industry or underfunding in diagnostic radiology, or both.

Deciding how much to spend

What cost effectiveness analysis cannot do is to help determine the *optimum* level of spending. It will not indicate whether too little or too much money is being spent, or in other words whether the doses being delivered to patients are higher or lower than what is reasonably achievable when social and *economic* factors are taken into account. This requires a method for comparing directly the benefits and the harm associated with different courses of action, which is an attribute of the widely used decision aiding technique known as cost–benefit analysis.

In cost–benefit analysis, both the total costs of implementing a method of dose reduction and the benefit derived from the reduced collective dose are expressed in monetary terms. If the costs exceed the benefit, then the protection method is not justified, since it will be attempting to reduce doses to below that which is reasonably achievable on economic grounds. In assessing the total costs, any concomitant degradation in the quality of the service provided by the medical exposure should be included as well as the financial costs of achieving the dose reduction, although it is usually difficult to quantify the former in monetary terms. Often the incremental cost effectiveness, discussed earlier, will provide a sufficient measure of the total costs per unit dose saved. It then remains to compare this with a monetary valuation of the benefit per unit dose saved, in order to determine whether the optimum level of protection has been reached.

Such a valuation, which is identical with that for the detriment per unit dose, is ultimately based on intrinsically controversial decisions regarding the value of changes in the life expectancy for unidentifiable individuals i.e. on the value of a premature statistical death. Following the human capital approach recommended by the NRPB, and accounting for the average life expectancy of patients who tend towards the elderly, a valuation of the harm associated with unit collective dose for use in general diagnostic radiology was estimated by Russell & Webb (1985) at between £5000 and £10000 per man Sv. (A value five times higher was suggested for paediatric and obstetric radiology because of the higher risk per unit dose for young patients and because of the promotion of parental anxiety.) Since this estimate was made, the perception of the cancer risk has increased and, more significantly, so has the Retail Price Index on which the valuation of the human capital losses from radiation-induced fatalities and genetic effects was based. These considerations have led to a 67% increase in the baseline value of the man Sv (Robb & Wrixon, 1988). Consequently, it would be more appropriate to take a figure of between £8000 and £17000 as the current (1991) value of a man Sv in adult diagnostic radiology, although the whole question is again under review by the NRPB.

Comparison of this value with those for incremental cost effectiveness listed in Table 13.2, demonstrates that for the hypothetical radiology department being illustrated, the costs of all the equipment modifications were well below the value of the benefit achieved. On purely radiological protection grounds, the implementation of all those equipment modifications would bring doses in that department closer to being as low as reasonably achievable (ALARA) and should therefore be carried out.

Similar cost–benefit comparisons have been made for other methods of reducing patient dose. It has been argued that even the high costs of replacing CT by MRI can be justified in terms of the greater saving in the cost of the potential radiation-induced cancers and genetic effects induced by CT that are totally avoided by use of MRI (Molyneux, 1991).

It should be stressed that, unless all the costs and benefits associated with different courses of action can be quantified in monetary terms, then cost–benefit analysis provides an incomplete assessment of the situation and should be regarded as only one input into decisions on health care spending. Other inputs may of necessity involve subjective judgments or the preferences of skilled medical and managerial professionals. It is possible to include these less quantifiable inputs in a formal decision aiding process by using a scoring system that weights options according to preferences. This is the essential feature of the technique known as multi-attribute utility analysis, which is discussed more fully in ICRP Publication 55 (ICRP 55, 1989).

Summary

The 1988 Ionising Radiation (POPUMET) Regulations call for adequate training in radiation protection for all those physically or clinically directing medical exposures. The Schedule to the Regulations outlines the requisite core of knowledge, which is covered point by point in the preceding chapters of this book.

However, radiologists and radiographers, no matter how well trained themselves, will always have difficulties in impressing upon hospital and health authority managers the need to devote scarce resources to improvements in radiological safety, because of the largely intangible benefits. The techniques for auditing the impact of radiation protection on the health care of patients outlined in this chapter can act as a powerful aid to investment decisions in an increasingly market oriented health service.

References

Croft, J. R. (1988). Optimisation of patient protection. In *Are X-rays Safe Enough? Patient Doses and Risks in Diagnostic Radiology*, ed. K. Faulkner & B. F. Wall, pp. 81–94. York: IPSM.

Fernandes-Russell, D., Bentham, G., Haynes, R., Kemp R. & Roberts, L. (1988). *The Economic Valuation of Statistical Life from Safety Assessment*. Research Report No. 5. Environmental Risk Assessment Unit. Norwich: University of East Anglia.

ICRP 26 (1977). *Recommendations of the International Commission on Radiological Protection*. ICRP Publication 26. Oxford: Pergamon Press.

ICRP 45 (1985). *Quantitative Bases for Developing a Unified Index of Harm*. ICRP Publication 45. Oxford: Pergamon Press.

ICRP 55 (1989). *Optimization and Decision-making in Radiological Protection*. ICRP Publication 55. Oxford: Pergamon Press.

ICRP 60 (1991). *1990 Recommendations of the International Commission on Radiological Protection*. ICRP Publication 60. Oxford: Pergamon Press.

Kind, P., Rosser, R. & Williams, A. (1982). Valuation of quality of life: some psychometric evidence. In *The Value of Life and Safety*, ed. M. W. Jones-Lee, pp. 159–170. Amsterdam: North Holland.

Molyneux, A. J. (1991). Computed tomography and radiation doses. *Lancet*, **337**, 1164.

NRPB (1990). Patient Dose Reduction in Diagnostic Radiology. *Documents of the NRPB*. Vol. 1, No. 3. London: HMSO.

Robb, J. D. & Wrixon, A. D. (1988). *Revised Estimates of the Monetary Value of Collective Dose*. NRPB-M157. Chilton: National Radiological Protection Board.

Russell, J. G. B. & Webb, G. A. M. (1985). Spending on radiation protection. *Lancet*, **1**, 391.

Wall, B. F. & Russell, J. G. B. (1988). The application of cost-utility analysis to radiological protection in diagnostic radiology. *Journal of Radiological Protection*, **8**, 221–9.

14

Dental radiography

J. SHEKHDAR

The use of dental X-ray equipment in the UK is subject to the following legislation:

1 The Ionising Radiations Regulations 1985.
2 The Ionising Radiation (POPUMET) Regulations 1988.

This legislation is supported in turn by the *Approved Code of Practice* (HSC, 1985) and by the *Guidance Notes* (NRPB, 1988).

In addition, the Department of Health have prepared some additional guidance notes designed specifically to assist in radiation protection matters relating to dental practice (DoH, 1990).

Introduction

Dental radiography is a high frequency, but low dose, technique. It contributes about 1% of the collective radiation dose to the UK population from diagnostic medical X-rays (NRPB, 1990*a*) (Fig. 14.1).

In 1981, 7.8 million dental X-ray examinations were carried out in the UK. Of these, approximately 6.7 million were intra-oral examinations (86%), 0.15 million were extra-oral (2%) and 0.91 million were pantomographic (12%).

Doses from different dental techniques have been measured by Wall & Kendall (1983). These results are listed in Table 14.1, together with a risk estimate. The dose is expressed as a weighted effective dose equivalent.

Together, these examinations give a collective dose of about 150 man Sv per year to the population of the UK. This is more than the entire collective dose resulting from the discharge of radioactive waste

Table 14.1. *Doses from different dental techniques*

Examination type	Dose (μSv)	Risk of fatal malignancy per million examinations[a]
Intra-oral (two films)	20	0.3
Extra-oral (two films)	30	0.5
Pantomographic (one film)	80	1.3

[a] Risk estimates are based on previous risk factors of 1.65% per Sv (see Wall & Kendall, 1983).

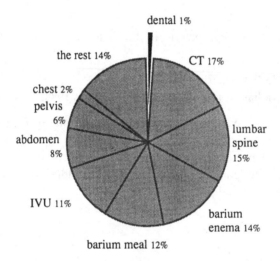

Fig. 14.1. The collective radiation dose to the UK population from medical diagnostic X-rays. Dental radiography accounts for about 1% of the total.

from hospitals, industry and the nuclear industry put together (NRPB, 1989).

Essential actions to meet legislative requirements

The requirements for the use of X-rays in dental work are similar to those for the use of X-rays in general diagnostic radiography:

1 The Health and Safety Executive must be notified of the use of X-rays.
2 An RPS (Radiation Protection Supervisor) must be appointed.
3 Local Rules must be provided.

4 The X-ray equipment must meet appropriate standards and must be checked and maintained regularly.
5 Contingency plans must be provided to describe the actions to be followed in the event of equipment malfunction.
6 Staff who are physically and clinically directing X-ray exposures must receive adequate training.
7 For dental work, an RPA (Radiation Protection Adviser) must be appointed, unless only the person undergoing the medical exposure is in the controlled area (defined as the area where the instantaneous dose rate exceeds 7.5 μSv/h). This is possible only if the requirements of the *Approved Code of Practice*, Part I, Paragraph 60 are complied with. These are:

1 Only one X-ray set (intra-oral/extra-oral or pantomographic) can be operated in a room at any one time.
2 The workload of the X-ray equipment does not exceed in any one week 30 mA min (dental radiography) or 150 mA min (panoramic tomography).
3 The X-ray set is of sound construction and properly maintained.

The extent of the controlled area will then be:

4 Within the primary beam until it has been sufficiently attenuated by distance or by absorption in material and in any direction within 1 m of the X-ray tube and 1 m of the patient.

When the X-ray equipment operates at or above 70 kV, the 1 m dimensions above should be increased to 1.5 m.

Local Rules
The Local Rules must contain:

1 The names of the employer, the RPA (if applicable) and the RPS.
2 The extent of the controlled areas around each X-ray set.
3 Written systems of work for any person, other than the patient who enters the controlled area.
4 Guidance on the use of the equipment to ensure that patient doses are kept as low as reasonably achievable.
5 Procedures to ensure that staff doses are kept as low as possible.

6 Instructions on the use of personal monitors if required.

7 Contingency plans and actions required if the X-ray exposure fails to terminate.

8 Instructions on the investigations to be carried out if a member of staff or a patient is exposed to ionising radiation to an extent significantly greater than intended.

It is also useful to list in an appendix the records that must be kept, namely the staff training records, equipment maintenance records, personal dosimetry records, checks of protective clothing, and quality control documentation.

A set of model Local Rules suitable for a dental practice is reproduced in Appendix C of the booklet *Radiation Protection in Dental Practice* (DoH, 1990).

Specific requirements for dental X-ray equipment

The requirements for equipment for dental radiography are given in Chapter 6 of the *Guidance Notes* (NRPB, 1988). Some of the requirements specific to dental equipment are outlined below:

1 The total filtration of the beam (inherent filtration of the X-ray tube plus any added filtration) must be equivalent to at least 1.5 mm of aluminium for X-ray tubes working up to voltages of 70 kV. At or above 70 kV, the filtration must comply with standards for general diagnostic radiography and must be equivalent to 2.5 mm of aluminium.

2 The voltage across the X-ray tube should not be less than 50 kV and preferably should be 70 kV.

3 Equipment used for intra-oral films must be fitted with a field-defining spacer cone. For equipment working at up to 60 kV, the cone must ensure a minimum focus-to-skin distance of 10 cm. For equipment working at higher voltages, the required distance is increased to 20 cm. The cone must also delineate the X-ray beam size, which must not exceed 6 cm at the patient's skin.

4 For panoramic tomography the beam size at the cassette holder should not exceed 10 mm × 150 mm.

5 Equipment used for cephalometry should have a means of confining the primary beam to the area of diagnostic interest.

6 There should be a visible indicator on the control panel to show that the set is in a state of readiness to produce X-rays. There

should also be a means of indicating to the operator that an exposure is taking place.

7 The exposure switch should be such that the exposure will continue only when pressure is maintained on the switch.

8 The cable to the switch should be at least 2 m long.

9 Equipment should be maintained regularly and a record kept of maintenance, faults and repairs.

10 A radiation survey should be carried out at least once every three years.

11 If a fault in the equipment occurs, then the equipment should be disconnected, labelled and the RPS should be informed.

12 Panoramic radiography must be stopped immediately if the rotational motion fails.

13 Intra-oral X-ray tubes, as used in intra-oral panoramic units, should be phased out as soon as practicable.

Limitations of patient dose

As is the case for general diagnostic radiography, radiation doses can be reduced most effectively by cutting out clinically unhelpful examinations. Existing films should be used wherever possible. Repeats due to incorrect X-ray exposures and film processing should be minimised. Higher radiation doses should never be given to compensate for poor film processing.

It can be seen from Table 14.1 that for a full mouth survey a lower radiation dose will be given by a pantomographic examination than by eight or more intra-oral films. Guidance on the use of pantomographic studies has been given by the Dental Practice Board (personal communication). The Board has stated that a panoral radiograph may be appropriate for a new patient to the practice, a patient for whom a comprehensive radiographic examination has not been done, and as an aid to examination when considering orthodontic treatment. A second panoral radiograph is not normally justified, but there are a few exceptions e.g. to follow up certain orthodontic treatments. It has to be said that these recommendations are based more on financial considerations than on those of radiation protection, but they are welcome, none the less.

In addition, the following points of technique should be noted:

1 The minimum number of films, consistent with adequate diagnosis, should be used.

2 The fastest film, consistent with good image quality, should be employed. Intensifying screens must be used for extra-oral and vertex occlusal views. Such screens should preferably be of the rare-earth type (Hutton *et al.*, 1987).

3 The smallest beam size practicable should be used. For intra-oral work, the field diameter must not exceed 6 cm. For paediatric pantomographic examinations, it may be possible to mask the top 15% of the collimating slit and reduce significantly the dose to the lens of the eye.

4 The beam should not be directed towards the gonads or the abdomen of women of reproductive age. If such a direction cannot be avoided, the patient's abdomen must be covered by a protective lead apron. Such lead aprons, of minimum lead equivalence 0.25 mm (NRPB, 1988), should be checked at least every 14 months.

5 The operator must check the exposure factors on each occasion before an examination is made. This is particularly important when there are interchangeable cones and field sizes.

Limitation of doses to staff and members of the public

Although not strictly relevant to radiation protection of the patient, there are a number of factors that relate to protection of the staff and the public:

1 Any person whose presence is unnecessary for the examination should be excluded from the X-ray room.

2 Operators must stand at least 2 m from the tube and patient. The lowest scatter doses for intra-oral work will be found at an angle between 90° and 150° from the direction of the primary beam (see Fig. 14.2).

3 A radiation warning sign is required on the door if the door opens straight into a controlled area. If the exposures can be of long duration (e.g. panoramic) a warning light or legend, which is lit automatically throughout the exposure, should be provided outside the door. The door must provide adequate shielding and be kept closed during radiography (NRPB, 1990*b*).

4 The X-ray unit should be disconnected from the mains electricity supply after use in order to de-designate the controlled area and eliminate the possibility of inadvertent exposure.

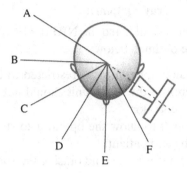

Dose rate at 0.5 m from phantom (mGy/h)

kVp(set)	A	B	C	D	E	F
50	3.6	0.7	0.4	1.1	3.2	5.0
60	8.3	1.8	1.1	1.8	5.8	9.0
70	16.2	3.6	2.5	3.2	8.6	13.2
80	27.4	5.8	4.3	1.4	13.0	19.0

Fig. 14.2. Measurements of scatter doses from a static dental unit. (Data courtesy of the Department of Medical Physics, Poole General Hospital.)

5 Staff must be monitored if the workload exceeds in 1 week:
   150 intra-oral films
   50 panoramic films (NRPB, 1988).
6 The operator should never hold the film, the patient or the tube housing during an exposure. If, for exceptional reasons, it is necessary to hold the film or to support a patient, an adult accompanying the patient should be asked to do so. The film should be held with forceps and protective gloves and lead aprons should be worn. Typical scatter doses per exposure from intra-oral films are:
   25 µSv to the hands 10 cm from the primary beam
   1 µSv to the body 50 cm from the primary beam.
   A member of the public must not receive a radiation dose to the body of greater than 1 mSv/year (in excess of background).
7 In cases where overexposure of the patient or a member of the public has occurred the incident must be investigated.

X-ray room design and siting of X-ray equipment

The requirements for room design are detailed in NRPB (1990*b*). Some of the main considerations are outlined below:

1 Access to the room during radiography must be restricted to the operator and the patient. Therefore the X-ray unit should not be installed in a waiting room or a corridor.
2 The room should be large enough to allow the operator to stand at least 2 m from the X-ray tube and patient.

   If this is not possible, the operator may stand outside the room provided that:

   1 During radiography, no-one can enter the room through another entrance.
   2 The patient can communicate easily with the operator.
   3 The audible warning can be heard and the exposure warning light can be observed as the operator approaches the controlled area on completion of an exposure.

   If these conditions cannot be fulfilled, then a protective screen must be provided. This must have attenuation properties to a lead equivalence of at least 1.25 mm. It must contain a viewing window of the same lead equivalence.

3 The equipment should be sited such that the operator can observe the patient, all entrances to the room and the exposure warning light. The primary beam should not be directed towards a door or window.
4 The room should offer adequate protection to persons in the adjacent areas. This will probably be the case if the room is built of solid construction materials (brick, concrete, high density blocks) and has solid floors.

   Additional shielding will be required if the main beam can point at a door, window or wall of lightweight construction. The lead equivalence required depends on the voltage used, but in practice the minimum available thickness of lead is 1.25 mm, which is quite adequate. When it can be guaranteed that only scattered radiation falls on a door, window or wall of light construction, extra shielding is unlikely to be needed, but there are exceptions.

   In certain circumstances, e.g. mobile caravans, it may be more

Table 14.2. *Results of a QA survey on 51 dental X-ray sets in the North-West Thames Region*

Survey result	Number
Total satisfactory	37 (73%)
Unsatisfactory	
Low filtration	9
Missing collimator	2
Incorrect cone	1
Mechanically unstable	2
Total unsatisfactory	14 (27%)
Total	51

practical to provide protection against the useful beam on only one wall and then adjust the position of the patient so that the X-ray beam can be directed at only that wall.

5 A mains supply switch should be readily accessible to the operator, preferably without passing through the controlled area.

Quality assurance in dental radiography

A regular programme of quality assurance is crucial to satisfactory radiography. For example, a survey of dental X-ray sets in the North-West Thames Region carried out in 1988 revealed major faults in about a quarter of the sets (Table 14.2).

The following points should be noted:

1 Equipment must be serviced regularly and a radiation survey carried out every three years.
2 Films must be stored correctly:

1 Films should not be stored in the room used for radiography. If this is not possible they should be in a lead box (at least 1.25 mm thick) and in an area of the room that receives scattered radiation only.
2 The humidity of the storage area should be between 30% and 50%, and the temperature between 10° and 20 °C.
3 Films should be used sequentially and not used after the expiry date.

3 Film processing:

1 The dark room should be light tight and fitted with the correct safelights.
2 Manual developing should be carried out at the recommended temperature and time. The influence of temperature is important, as the following figures show (from a widely used manufacturer of dental photographic supplies):

Temperature (°C)	Development time (min)
20	5
21	4.5
22	4

A thermometer (not mercury) and a stopwatch must be provided. The developer should be renewed at least once per month.
3 For automatic processing, the temperature and replenishment rates should be checked regularly and, if necessary, adjusted to those recommended. The rollers should be cleaned regularly.
4 The dates of the solution changes (or replenishment rates) and the solution temperature should be recorded.

An assessment of film processing at 11 dental clinics in the North-West Thames Region showed only three systems to be working properly: three of the processed films were so badly fogged that they were unreadable, and five others were significantly underdeveloped.

Summary

Dental radiography must comply with the same regulations with which conventional radiography complies. Radiation doses to individual patients are low but, because of the large number of patients X-rayed, the collective dose to the population is not negligible. Care in siting and regular maintenance of the equipment will reduce doses to both staff and patients. To produce X-ray films with a good image quality using a low radiation dose requires attention to film processing; this is often a neglected area.

References

DoH (1990). *Radiation Protection in Dental Practice*. London: DoH.

The Ionising Radiations Regulations 1985. Statutory Instrument No. 1333. London: HMSO.

The Ionising Radiation (Protection of Persons Undergoing Medical Examination or Treatment) Regulations 1988. Statutory Instrument No. 778. London: HMSO.

HSC (1985). *Approved Code of Practice. The Protection of Persons Against Ionising Radiation Arising from any Work Activity*. London: HMSO.

Hutton, J. B., Brennan, A. G. & Bird P. D. (1987). Dose reduction in lateral cephalometry using rare-earth screens. *British Dental Journal*, **163**, 378–82.

NRPB (1988). *Guidance Notes for the Protection of Persons Against Ionising Radiations Arising from Medical and Dental Use*. London: HMSO.

NRPB (1989). *Radiation Exposure of the UK Population – 1988 Review*. NRPB-R227. London: HMSO.

NRPB (1990*a*). Patient Dose Reduction in Diagnostic Radiology. *Documents of the NRPB*. Vol. 1, No. 3, London: HMSO.

NRPB (1990*b*). *Advice to Dental Equipment Companies – Location of Dental X-ray Equipment*. NRPB DMS-M3. Leeds: NRPB.

Wall, B. F. & Kendall, G. M. (1983). Collective doses and risks from dental radiology in Great Britain. *British Journal of Radiology*, **56**, 511–6.

15

Cardiology and orthopaedic work

M. WEST

Mobile image intensifier equipment

Special problems of radiation protection, concerning both patient and operator, arise with the use of mobile image intensifier equipment. The majority of such work can be divided into two distinct categories:

1 Orthopaedic work in an operating theatre, using X-ray equipment with a C-arm configuration.
2 Cardiac pacemaker wire insertions, using a C-arm unit or equipment with a linear image intensifier movement.

Orthopaedics

In order that the mobile X-ray equipment should be small and easy to manoeuvre, major components such as the X-ray tube and the image intensifier are designed to be as small as possible. The imaging capabilities of this mobile equipment are, therefore, considerably less than those of a conventional fluoroscopy unit. The problem is exacerbated by the variable geometry of the C-arm support of the X-ray unit, which demands accurate alignment to produce the required image projection. These factors combine to reduce the margin for error in producing acceptable images and can lead to prolonged examinations and unnecessarily high patient radiation doses.

Experience of this particular problem in the North-West Thames Region indicates that significant improvements in image quality and patient dose reduction can be achieved if the X-ray equipment is operated by an *experienced* radiographer with a good practical knowledge of theatre imaging techniques.

In general, the production of high quality fluoroscopic images under theatre conditions places far greater technical demands on the operator than does conventional fluoroscopy.

Cardiology

When a temporary, or permanent, pacemaker wire insertion is carried out with mobile X-ray equipment it is essential that a *dedicated*, *radiolucent* patient table is used. The use of patient supports with a higher attenuation, or even of standard beds, will lead to poor image quality, increased patient dose and a reduction in X-ray tube life.

As in any fluoroscopic examination, the exposure time should be

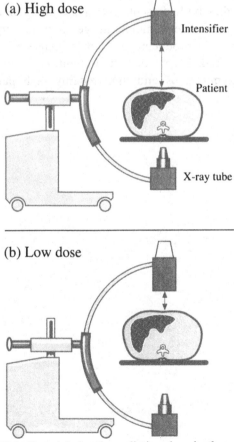

(a) High dose

Intensifier

Patient

X-ray tube

(b) Low dose

Fig. 15.1. To minimise the radiation dose in the case of mobile image intensifier equipment, the intensifier should be as close as possible to the patient.

kept to a minimum, but particular attention should be paid to *minimising the patient–image intensifier separation* as a method of reducing the patient radiation dose. This is relatively straightforward when using an X-ray system with a linear intensifier movement, since the X-ray tube–intensifier distance can be varied to bring the intensifier as close to the patient as practicable. A unit with a C-arm configuration, however, will have a fixed X-ray tube–intensifier distance and so the patient must be raised to the required height. This means that the patient table must not only be radiolucent, but also capable of elevating the patient (Fig. 15.1).

Summary

Cardiology and orthopaedics both present special problems of radiation protection because of the use of mobile image intensifier equipment. The margin for error in producing acceptable images is much lower than in conventional radiography and strict attention to detail is required if prolonged examinations and unnecessarily high patient doses are to be avoided.

Appendix. Making the best use of a department of radiology

ROYAL COLLEGE OF RADIOLOGISTS

Adapted from: *Making the best use of a Department of Radiology: Guidelines for Doctors*
RCR Working Party (1989), Royal College of Radiologists, London

The following guidelines have been designed to help hospital doctors and general practitioners make the best use of their local X-ray Department. **The guidelines are not intended to replace clinical judgement but to support it in times of doubt or difficulty.** Recently introduced legislation (*Ionising Radiations* 1988) requires those responsible for the provision and use of radiation to comply with guidelines of good practice.

In these guidelines, requests for X-rays have been separated into three categories: 'selective'; 'routine'; and 'screening'. Uninformed or uncritical use of X-ray examinations either as part of a routine practice or as screening tests is the greatest source of unnecessary use at the present time.

The 'selective' request

When a patient has signs and symptoms suggestive of a particular pathology or disease and **radiology is used to confirm the diagnosis,** then the X-ray examination is used selectively.

For example hip tenderness in an elderly patient who is also unable to weight bear following a fall suggests a fracture of the femur; a diagnosis which can be confirmed by X-ray examination.

The 'routine' request

In many diagnostic situations circumstantial, as opposed to symptomatic, evidence of a particular disease has become accepted as sufficient to generate strong suspicion. If an X-ray examination is used to confirm or refute such suspicion, then it is said to be used 'routinely'.

An example is the routine use of intravenous urography in hypertensive patients who have no signs or symptoms of urinary tract disease. When the disease occurs only very infrequently, **so that the association between the circumstantial evidence and the disease is weak** (as in the above example) routine radiological examination cannot be justified.

The 'screening' request

When a patient is well and **has no signs or symptoms suggesting the presence of a disorder which radiography might reveal** then the X-ray examination is used as a screening test.

For example, use of the chest X-ray to screen for lung cancer, or as a pre-employment examination in a person with no signs or symptoms of respiratory disease. Apart from certain exceptional circumstances such requests should be actively discouraged.

Balancing the likely costs and benefits

When requesting any radiological investigation you should bear in mind that all X-rays are potentially carcinogenic and teratogenic.

The patient's interest will only be best served if the likely costs of the examination (inconvenience, discomfort, the risk of radiation to those X-rayed, and the benefits which might have to be foregone when resources are committed to the X-ray examination) are less than the anticipated benefits.

Many of the guidelines presented here are based on formal studies of these issues as applied to specific radiological procedures used in particular clinical circumstances.

The medico-legal position

Such is the perceived risk of medical litigation that X-rays are sometimes requested even when they are not considered clinically necessary by the requesting doctor. If, as a result of careful clinical examination, you decide that an X-ray is not necessary for the future management of the patient, your decision is unlikely to be challenged on medico-legal grounds but do remember to record the results of your clinical examination in the patient's notes.

Should you decide to follow the guidelines described here, your position will be further strengthened because it will have the support of the Royal College of Radiologists.

Your relationship with the department of radiology

Request forms should be completed accurately and legibly in order to avoid any misinterpretation. You should state clearly the reasons for the request and give sufficient clinical details to enable the radiologist to understand the particular problems that you are attempting to resolve by X-ray examination.

If you are in doubt as to whether an investigation is required or which investigation is best, it makes sense to ask the radiologist who, like other consultants, will know much more about his or her specialty than those whose primary interests are more general.

The pregnant patient

Irradiation of any area from the diaphragm to the knees should be avoided in early pregnancy unless there are overriding clinical considerations. You as the referring clinician have the prime responsibility to avoid unnecessary irradiation of a fetus. If the patient is, or might be, pregnant the department of radiology must be informed.

If in doubt, you should contact a consultant radiologist who may suggest an alternative type of examination.

How to interpret the guidelines

The following lists present guidelines on **12 types of X-ray examination** which together comprise some 95% of radiological practice in NHS hospitals.

Guidance for selecting patients for a particular X-ray examination is laid out in three columns. **The first column lists the more common circumstances** in which the examination is currently used. The majority of entries under this heading are clinical and refer to the patient's presenting symptoms and signs. Non clinical circumstances of examination use, for example pre-employment chest X-ray, are listed next.

Additional guidelines specifically for use with children will be found at the end of each list of examination circumstances.

In the second column you will find the guideline which should generally govern the use of the X-ray examination in the adjacent circumstance. **The third column lists any better known and generally agreed exceptions** to the guideline.

Guidelines and exceptions can always be waived at your discretion but, if you do this, it would be helpful to the radiologist and for the guideline review process if you could state your reasons for doing so on the X-ray request form.

Example 1

Should an asymptomatic 35 year old man admitted to hospital for a routine herniorrhaphy have a pre-operative chest X-ray?

Look up **procedure – chest X-ray** [on p. 135] then the **circumstance** pre-operation; **guideline** – chest X-ray not recommended; **exception** – cardiopulmonary surgery.

Example 2

Should a chest X-ray be taken following the aspiration of a pleural effusion?

Look up **procedure – chest X-ray** [on p. 135] then the **circumstance** – pleural effusion; **guideline** – a chest X-ray after aspiration of a pleural effusion rarely provides useful information; **exception** – a deterioration in the patient's condition.

Example 3

A 60 year old man attends the accident and emergency unit following a head injury with a history of brief loss of consciousness (five minutes). The clinical examination is normal. Should a skull X-ray be requested?

Look up **procedure** – **skull X-ray** [on p. 138] then the **circumstance** – head injury; **guideline** – skull X-ray is not recommended routinely; **exception** – selective use is recommended in the presence of a loss of consciousness, however brief, since injury.

(Note – In this example there are several other exceptions to the guideline.)

The Guidelines

Chest X-ray

Circumstance	Guidelines	Exceptions
Active systemic disease	Selective X-ray recommended depending on clinical indications rather than routinely according to a time schedule.	
Cardiovascular disease	Fluoroscopy of the heart to detect inert ventricular segments is of no value. Assessment of cardiac chamber enlargement by chest radiography with barium swallow is an outmoded form of investigation.	
Malignant disease known to be present – bronchus and other sites	Selective X-ray recommended depending on clinical indications rather than routinely according to a time schedule.	
Non-specific ill health	In the absence of fever or respiratory symptoms, it is unlikely that an X-ray will produce evidence of significant chest disease in patients of any age.	Guidelines may be waived at the discretion of the clinician e.g. if clinical examination suggests that malignancy or pulmonary tuberculosis is a definite possibility.
Pleural effusion – after aspiration	A chest radiograph rarely provides useful information.	A deterioration in the patient's clinical condition.
Pleural effusion/ consolidation	Tomography of the hilar region is rarely helpful in the presence of a pleural effusion (or adjacent consolidation). Bronchoscopy is likely to be of more value.	
Pulmonary disease – chronic obstructive	Useful for initial confirmation but not helpful in follow-up.	If disease severe, or if repeated attacks, or if sudden deterioration e.g. asthma.

Chest X-ray (*cont.*)

Circumstance	Guidelines	Exceptions
Pulmonary oedema	Useful for initial confirmation of diagnosis. Response to treatment can often be assessed clinically.	Repeat only if deterioration in patient's clinical condition
Reactions to certain specific treatments such as immunosuppressive therapy, chemotherapy or radiotherapy	Projections other than a postero-anterior (PA) film are rarely indicated.	
Post surgery/ thoracotomy	Post-operative radiographs should be restricted to patients in whom there is difficulty managing tubes, drains and ventilation; **or if** there is significant change in the patient's clinical condition.	
Respiratory tract infection – lower	Can be useful for establishing initial diagnosis.	Selective investigation recommended in presence of specific indications such as suspected or known tuberculosis, deterioration in patient's condition and failure to respond to treatment. Selective radiography to confirm that lower respiratory tract infection has cleared following treatment may be needed in middle aged and elderly patients, particularly in those who smoke.
Respiratory tract infection – upper	Not recommended.	

Indication	Not indicated	Indicated
Trauma to chest	Routine demonstration of simple rib fracture in minor trauma is not recommended.	Severe trauma, particularly a deceleration injury; suspected multiple fractures; suspected pleural or pulmonary injury.
To screen for bronchial carcinoma	Not recommended. Periodic X-rays to detect early lung cancer do not influence the prognosis.	
To screen for pulmonary tuberculosis	Not recommended routinely.	When the incidence of pulmonary tuberculosis in the patient's ethnic group may be more than 1:1000 and when chest X-ray has not been performed within the last six months.
Pre-operation	Not recommended.	Cardiopulmonary surgery; if clinical examination suggests that malignancy or pulmonary tuberculosis is a strong possibility; when the incidence of pulmonary tuberculosis in the patient's ethnic group may be more than 1:1000 and when chest X-ray has not been performed within the last six months.
On admission to hospital, during pregnancy, pre-employment	Not recommended.	Guidelines may be waived at the discretion of the clinician e.g. if clinical examination suggests that malignancy or pulmonary tuberculosis is a strong possibility.
Chest infection (children)	Frequent follow-up films are unnecessary. A baseline chest radiograph is all that is required.	A deterioration in the child's clinical condition.

Chest X-rays account for **33%** of all examinations.

Skull X-ray

Circumstance	Guidelines	Exceptions
Cerebral symptoms **with** focal signs or symptoms	A lateral radiograph is all that is necessary in most cases.	Other views may be required to localise an area of calcification.
Cerebral symptoms **without** focal signs or symptoms	Not recommended routinely.	

Head injury	Not recommended routinely.	Selective X-ray is recommended in the presence of any of the following:
		• suspected skull penetration or foreign body
		• patients who present with any of the following signs or symptoms:
		  – CSF and/or blood discharge from the nose
		  – haemotympanum and/or blood discharge from the ear
		  – loss of consciousness, however brief, since injury
		  – other focal signs or symptoms
		• head injury plus other trauma (e.g. broken limbs) which might imply a particularly strong force of impact
		• possible head injury in the presence of additional pathological findings (e.g. stroke, epileptic seizure, mental handicap) which might preclude a proper clinical examination
		
		Additional Note
		Those who live alone or in a domestic situation which precludes proper surveillance of the patient's condition over the following seven days should be admitted for observation rather than sent home on the basis of a negative skull X-ray.

	Guidelines	Exceptions
Head injury **with alcoholic intoxication** which may prevent proper clinical examination	X-ray may be helpful **but only if** the patient's condition will allow the taking of films of diagnostic quality. Otherwise admission for observation may sometimes be preferable.	
Epilepsy (children)	Not recommended routinely.	
Head injury (children)	Not recommended routinely.	Selective use as for adults [see p. 138]
Sinusitis (children)	Sinuses poorly developed under 6–9 years. Radiographs are of limited value in this age group.	

Skull X-rays account for **8%** of all examinations.

X-ray of lumbar spine

Circumstance	Guidelines	Exceptions
Back pain	Not recommended routinely. Acute back pain is usually due to conditions which cannot be diagnosed by plain film radiography. Pain correlates poorly with the severity of degenerative change found on radiology.	Symptoms getting worse, or not resolving; neurological signs; or a history of trauma.
Asymptomatic patients e.g. pre-employment screening	Not recommended. There is no correlation between radiological findings and likelihood of future disability.	

X-rays of the spine account for 9% of all examinations

X-ray of cervical spine

Circumstance	Guidelines	Exceptions
Neck pain	Not recommended. Acute neck pain is usually due to conditions which cannot be diagnosed by plain film radiography. Pain correlates poorly with the severity of degenerative change found on radiology.	Symptoms getting worse, or not resolving; neurological signs; or a history of trauma.

X-ray of thoracic spine

Circumstance	Guidelines	Exceptions
Back pain	Not recommended. Degenerative changes are almost universal in middle age onwards. Assessing their clinical significance is often impossible.	Localised pain and tenderness; root pain; long tract signs with a sensory level; or known primary malignant disease.

X-rays of the spine account for **9%** of all examinations.

X-ray of limbs and joints

Circumstance	Guidelines	Exceptions
Inflammatory joint disease	May be useful as part of initial assessment but follow-up films are rarely helpful.	When an operation is contemplated.
Injury	Selective X-ray is recommended in patients presenting with one or more of following: • signs of fracture such as deformity, crepitus or instability • bruising or severe swelling • moderate to severe pain on weight bearing • point tenderness on palpation • any positive sign in a knee • injury of tendon, vessel or nerve • suspected foreign body	
Skeletal metastases suspected	An isotope scan should be the initial investigation in patients with suspected skeletal metastases; and in patients who may be developing osteomyelitis (especially those with a predisposing factor such as sickle cell disease or ethnic susceptibility).	
Skeletal trauma (children)	X-ray of the contra-lateral side, for comparison, is unnecessary as a routine.	In exceptional circumstances where there is strong clinical evidence of a fracture but no apparent radiographic evidence, films of the contra-lateral side **may** be useful e.g. to show avulsion of a medial humeral epicondyle.
Spina bifida occulta suspected in children with sacral dimple	Not recommended.	

X-rays of limbs and joints account for **34%** of all examinations.

Plain abdominal X-ray

Circumstance	Guidelines	Exceptions
Abdominal trauma	An erect chest film to demonstrate disease above the abdomen is recommended in addition to a supine abdominal film. **If** intestinal obstruction or perforation suspected, an erect (or lateral decubitus) abdominal film is also recommended. **If** abdominal X-rays are normal but there is still a strong clinical suspicion of organ rupture discuss further investigation with a radiologist.	
Acute abdominal pain	An erect chest film to demonstrate disease above the abdomen is recommended in addition to a supine abdominal film. **If** intestinal obstruction or perforation suspected, an erect abdominal film is also recommended.	
Gall stones suspected	Plain films of the right upper quadrant with ultrasound examination are recommended. **If** calculi are demonstrated, no further imaging investigation is required [see p. 147].	Cholecystography is recommended if ultrasound is not immediately available.
Haematemesis and/or melaena	Not recommended [see p. 144].	
Lost intra-uterine contraceptive device (IUCD)	Ultrasound is the examination of choice.	Plain films, AP and lateral of pelvis, are indicated if IUCD not localised on ultrasound examination.

Renal colic	A plain film may show calculi but intravenous urography is the definitive investigation. Discuss with radiologist.
Renal size assessment	Plain films usually unhelpful. Ultrasound is the examination of choice.
Intestinal obstruction (neonates)	An inversion view in neonates with anorectal atresia is not recommended as it does not affect early management.
Intussusception (children)	Supine and erect abdominal films recommended [see p. 146].

Barium examination of oesophagus, stomach and duodenum

Circumstance	Guidelines	Exceptions
Duodenal ulcer – follow-up	Not recommended.	
Dyspepsia and additional signs suggesting peptic ulcer or carcinoma	Double contrast barium meal or endoscopy may be the initial investigation depending on local availability.	
Dysphagia	Barium swallow is the recommended intitial investigation.	
Gastric outlet obstruction suspected	Endoscopy preferred. Otherwise gastric lavage and decompression should be performed before attempting a barium meal.	
Gastric ulcer – follow-up to assess healing	Endoscopy is recommended.	
Gastrointestinal bleeding – acute upper	Not recommended. Endoscopy is the preferred method of investigation.	
Pancreatic or biliary disease suspected	Not recommended. Endoscopy, ultrasound or CT preferable.	
Resected stomach – assessment of	Not recommended. Endoscopy is the preferred method of investigation.	
Bile-stained vomiting suggesting mal-rotation (children)	Recommended to confirm mal-rotation of the duodenum.	

Barium examination of small bowel

A small bowel examination should not be regarded as a continuation of a barium meal examination of the stomach and duodenum but as a separate procedure for which there are several techniques, some involving duodenal intubation.

Circumstance	Guidelines	Exceptions
Intestinal blood loss, chronic or recurrent, presenting as anaemia	Recommended.	
Malabsorption	Recommended particularly when other non-radiological investigations such as small bowel biopsy are normal.	
Small bowel disease suspected e.g. Crohn's disease	Small bowel studies are recommended. Findings can be useful for diagnosis and both short and long-term management.	
Small bowel obstruction – acute	Not recommended. Small bowel series rarely give more information than plain abdominal films.	
Small bowel obstruction – chronic	Small bowel studies are recommended. Findings can be useful for diagnosis and both short and long-term management.	

Barium examination of large bowel

Circumstance	Guidelines	Exceptions
Inflammatory bowel disease or tumour suggested by abdominal pain, rectal bleeding or change in bowel habit	Double contrast barium enema is recommended **but only** after rectal examination and sigmoidoscopy followed by full bowel preparation.	Toxic megacolon is an **absolute contra-indication** for this examination. If rectal/colon biopsy using a rigid sigmoidoscope has been performed in the previous seven days, or in the case of a fibreoptic endoscope in the previous two days, then the examination should be delayed.
Large bowel obstruction – acute	A limited single contrast study is recommended under certain circumstances but only after consultation and review of plain films with a radiologist.	
Ulcerative colitis – acute exacerbation	Bowel preparation for double contrast barium enema should be avoided if severe inflammatory disease is suspected.	Under certain circumstances a limited enema without prior bowel preparation is recommended but **discuss with radiologist first.**
Ulcerative colitis or polyp(s) – long term follow-up	Double contrast barium enema recommended.	See guideline above for 'acute exacerbation'.
Entero-colitis – necrotising (children)	A contrast examination is not recommended in the acute phase.	

Circumstance	Guidelines	Exceptions
Intussusception (children)	Diagnostic and therapeutic barium enema recommended.	Signs of peritonism, free gas on the plain films and a shocked child are contra-indications which require consultation with the surgeon and radiologist before investigation.
Rectal bleeding (children)	Isotope scan should be initial investigation to look for Meckel's diverticulum.	Request a barium enema if the isotope scan is negative.

Examination of the biliary tract

Circumstance	Guidelines	Exceptions
Gall stones or cholecystitis suspected	Where ultrasound is available it is the first choice investigation. Otherwise plain films of the abdomen are recommended [see p. 142]. If no opaque calculi are found, an oral cholecystogram is the recommended investigation.	
Jaundice – obstructive with or without suspicion of gall stones	Ultrasound examination is recommended. Discuss findings and possible further investigation with a radiologist.	

Examination of the urinary tract

Circumstance	Guidelines	Exceptions
Haematuria	Intravenous urography is recommended. If the result is normal discuss further investigation with a radiologist.	
Hypertension with no other evidence of urinary disease	Intravenous urography not recommended. Discuss alternative investigation with a radiologist.	Hypertension in young adults or in others not well controlled by medication.
Renal colic	A plain film may show calculi but intravenous urography is the definitive investigation. Discuss with a radiologist.	
Urinary retention	Ultrasound examination of the urinary tract is the investigation of choice. Intravenous urography not recommended.	
Urinary tract infection, recurrent (young women)	Intravenous urography not recommended routinely.	Selective use of intravenous urography may be helpful if additional factors such as: haematuria, previous acute pyelonephritis, childhood urinary tract infection, history of calculi or obstruction, raised serum creatinine, previous genito-urinary surgery, or severe diabetes mellitus are present.
Enuresis – persisting (children)	Ultrasound recommended. If abnormal or ultrasound not available, proceed to intravenous urography.	
Urinary tract infection (children)	Follow local policy. A nationally agreed approach to investigation is not yet available.	

Index